HOT
PLANTS

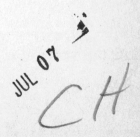

JUL 07

CH

ALSO BY CHRIS KILHAM

Psyche Delicacies
Tales from the Medicine Trail
Kava, Medicine Hunting in Paradise
The Five Tibetans

CHRIS KILHAM

HOT PLANTS

Nature's Proven Sex Boosters
for Men and Women

ST. MARTIN'S GRIFFIN

NEW YORK

www.stmartins.com

ISBN 0-312-31539-2
EAN 978-0312-31539-9

First published in the United States by St. Martin's Griffin

10 9 8 7 6 5 4 3 2

To Maria Sena, the shaman's shaman, who pointed a bony finger at me and said, "You bridge the worlds." Thank you for your wisdom, insight, and spirit.

IMPORTANT NOTE
TO READERS

The material in this book is for informational purposes only. It is not intended to diagnose, treat, or serve as a prescription for any illness or disease, or to replace the advice of your medical doctor. If you suffer from any medical conditions, please see your physician before following any of the suggestions in this book.

The material in this book is intended to support healthy sexual function and enjoyment. Please keep in mind that practicing safer sex and preventing sexually transmitted diseases are important practices for anyone who is sexually active.

The fact that a Web site or other source is listed in this book as a potential source of information does not mean that my publisher or I endorses any of the information or recommendations that source may provide. Likewise, the fact that my own Web site is listed does not mean that my publisher endorses any of the information or recommendations that my site may provide. Finally, the fact that my own products are listed does not mean that my publisher endorses them.

CONTENTS

ACKNOWLEDGMENTS

IT IS SIMPLY NOT FEASIBLE TO THANK EVERYBODY WHO HAS helped me in the research and writing of this book; the people in that category are legion. I wish to acknowledge Natalie and Paul Koether, without whose remarkable support I would not have been able to pursue my research to the extent that I have for the past nine years. Thanks also to Mel Rich, who has supported several of my ventures. Thanks to Annie Eng for being a fabulous help and traveling companion in Malaysia; to Marat Khamzin and Vadim Kolpakov for their kind support in Siberia; to shaman Bernie Peixoto (Ipupiara) for his companionship and guidance in the Brazilian Amazon; to Jerry Wu and his crew in southeastern China; to Craig Weatherby and Muhammed Majeed for tremendous assistance in my Indian research; to Dr. Quaynor for his help in Ghana; to Travis Hammond and Lieutenant Elias Faraoun for help in Lebanon and Syria; for Sergio Cam and his Chakarunas crew in the Peruvian highlands; to Gordon and Xiao Nan Gray for their guidance in Heilongjiang; to Zachary and Hanna Gibson for support in Hawaii; to Kenneth Miller for a fabulous assist in Venezuela; to Country

Girl for company here in the hills; and to Lyle Craker and Zoe Gardner for support at U Mass, Amherst. Thanks to my agent, Anne Sellaro, and my editor, Diane Reverand, at St. Martin's Press. Many hundreds of others have helped me as well, providing guidance, assistance of all kinds, generous hospitality, and good humor, and have shared the mind-opening, boundary-blurring times and circumstances that arise on the medicine trail.

I salute you all.

—Chris Kilham

FOREWORD

ON A SUNNY MARCH MORNING, I FOUND MYSELF, AT AGE SIX-
teen, walking alone along a quaint cobblestone street some-
where in old San Juan, Puerto Rico. I could smell the sea and
hear birds chirping and warbling gaily from roofs and wires.
The day matched my enthusiasm and *grand sense of delight*.
Later, friends informed me that the area was highly dangerous. I
could only shrug at the news. Sometimes fate favors the bliss-
fully naïve. I encountered no trouble.

As I strode along in happy reverie, I heard the percussive
clacking of castanets above me. Looking up to the source, I es-
pied a balcony, where a statuesque raven-haired beauty stood at
a wrought-iron railing, gazing at me through dark, mischievous
eyes. Her shining tresses were pulled back and adorned with a
fresh hibiscus blossom behind one ear. Her wide, sumptuous
lips were painted a vivid carmine, and I caught the flicker of a
tongue tip snaking along the ridge of her upper teeth. She wore
a purfled dress of red and black, and black high-heeled boots
that laced to the knee. The golden light of late morning slanted
from atop the building across the street, capturing her like

a spotlight. I felt way out of my depth. A man could fall hard for a woman like that, like a grand piano pushed off a roof.

She raised her head in a suggestive greeting, as one castaneted hand described a circle, summoning me up to join her. A smile crept across her face, and her voluptuous mouth opened wider. One eyebrow lifted, she waited for an answer. I swallowed hard, took a breath, and cast a more careful look around. Between the woman and myself was a narrow and dark staircase that led up into a yellow stucco building to the floor where she stood. I had no way to tell what waited for me on the stairs. How I wanted to rise up into the air, touch down in front of her, and lose myself in her. But all my instincts told me to forget the idea. I exhaled to let out pressure, gave a friendly and regretful smile, and took my leave with a wave good-bye.

Moments like that linger in the mind, casting a long shadow over the years that follow, teasing the reptilian brain, tickling the nerves, and cooing from memory's dark alleys on certain moon-lit nights. So, too, like the sultry siren on the balcony in old San Juan, the hot plants have summoned me suggestively, as I have wended my way from one continent to another in an ongoing quest for nature's cures.

As a medicine hunter, I spend much of my time scouring the jungles, mountains, forests, valleys, and remote parts of the world, seeking out healing plants from all traditions. In my travels along the medicine trail to the Amazon, China, India, Siberia, Africa, the South Pacific, the Middle East, Thailand, Malaysia, Europe, and numerous ports of call, the hot plants have called to me like that woman on the balcony. They have summoned me from fields of high grasses and on windy mountain slopes. I have heard intriguing tales of their powers in markets and on forest trails, and sitting around late-night fires. Men and women have brought them to me and offered them in cupped hands. They have told me their stories and have shared the secrets of plants, which stir the juices of our sexual desires as surely as fire heats a pot.

A curious string of events, one after another, year by year, spanning decades now, has equipped me with a broad knowledge of these plants. All in all, it has been a strange and marvelous adventure.

Even as tales of the hot plants have come to me by unusual means, scientists in laboratories and research facilities worldwide have probed into the precise chemical nature and bodily effects of these plants. I have been fortunate to sit with some of the preeminent scientists working with the hot plants. The same bitter tree bark that I have sampled in some damp jungle has become the object of scrutiny in a sanitary research facility. I have sat with shamans who possess expert knowledge of these sex enhancers, while today physicians are administering modern standardized dosages of the hot plants to patients with good results.

As a faculty member at a major educational institution, the University of Massachusetts at Amherst, I know very well that expertise in the field and in the lab is essential to complete understanding of any beneficial plant, though I would rather spend my days tramping through the forest than staring into a microscope or taking blood samples in a clinic. In these pages I share with you the work that goes on in both places. From forest to lab, from field to finished products, the hot plants have come of age and are available to enhance your sex life. And I am delighted to introduce you to these extraordinary botanicals.

These hot plants are not only nature's sure-fire agents of sexual desire and function; their existence is vital proof that for every need, nature provides an answer. For every desire, nature possesses an agent to enhance that desire, and to lead to its fulfillment. When you choose to employ them, you will know their effectiveness firsthand. I invite you to join me along the medicine trail, to learn the secrets of the hot plants for yourself.

Chris Kilham
Western Massachusetts
2004

INTRODUCTION:
NATURE'S AGENTS OF
DESIRE

IN OUR JOURNEY TOGETHER THROUGH THE WORLD OF HOT
plants, I will take you to the Amazon, Africa, China, India,
Malaysia, Siberia, the Middle East, and other lands. As we
travel, I will introduce you to the most effective sex enhancing
plants. If you believe that nature offers no true aphrodisiacs,
and that only pharmaceutical drugs can enhance your sex life,
the guide you hold in your hands will convince you otherwise.
You will find yourself liberated from a notion that is at best in-
correct, and at worst conspiratorial. If you accept that nature
with its miraculous diversity offers love and sex potions of various types, this book will help you to know them, find them,
and use them. The resource section at the end of this book will
give you valuable information for leading a more sexually vital,
satisfied life.

We may never know when people first employed plants to
enhance their sexual desire, function, or satisfaction, but we do
know that the human use of plants for health purposes dates
back a very long time. Neanderthals lived from about 200,000
years ago until roughly 30,000 years ago in Europe and western

Asia. They coexisted with modern humans for most of the period but then mysteriously vanished. Physical evidence of the use of plant remedies goes back some 60,000 years to a burial site at Shanidar Cave, Iraq, in which a Neanderthal man was uncovered in 1960. He had been buried with eight species of plants, seven of which are still used for medicinal purposes today.

The Shanidar Neanderthal isn't the only dead man to achieve celebrity in modern medicinal circles. On September 19, 1991, an extraordinary discovery took place in Austria's Otzal Alps, when two hikers came upon an ice mummy preserved by freezing. The analysis of samples of organic tissues has determined that the "Iceman" lived between 3350 and 3100 B.C. and died approximately 5,200 years ago. At death he was between forty and fifty years old, and he appears to have suffered from a number of medical conditions. He turned into a mummy by chance, due to freezing weather conditions. The Iceman's possessions have given scientists a better look at what life was like during the Neolithic Age in Europe. Perhaps the most valuable possession, according to many scientists, was his "medicine kit." The Iceman wore on his left wrist two walnut-sized pieces of birch fungus, drilled through the middle and held in place with twisted fur strips. Also known as Chaga (*Inonotus obliquus*), the fungus is antibiotic and is known by modern science to be highly active against some types of mycobacteria such as tuberculosis. I have researched Chaga in Siberia, where it has been studied for its anticancer properties.

Humanity's relationship with plants is intimate and ongoing. We have coevolved with plants since the earliest stages of our origins, deep in the murky, primordial swamp of biological prehistory. Ingredients in plants, from carbohydrates, fats, and proteins to vitamins and minerals, are integral to our body composition and chemistry. Indeed, our very lives depend on the nutrients provided by the plant kingdom. Some compounds perform the same functions in plants and in our bodies. Natural antioxidant phenols in plants, for example, protect plant cells from oxidation and often offer the same protective function for our cells. Our bodies know the substances that occur in plants. We are biologically familiar with plant compounds and possess an innate capacity to metabolize and utilize those compounds, whether they are vitamins, carbohydrates, or curative agents.

We eat plants, drink their juices, wear their fibers, color with their dyes, build homes with materials derived from them, employ them as medicines, and use them to enhance our life experience in a variety of ways. We distill essences from them to create evocative scents. We consume an extraordinary array of aromatic spices, from pungent to sweet. We also employ a select number of very special plants to enhance sex. We always have and always will use these hot plants.

For our purposes, the interchangeable terms *herb, botanical,* or *plant remedy* refer to any and all flora or parts of them, including grasses, flowers, berries, seeds, leaves, nuts, stems, stalks, and roots, which are used for their therapeutic and health-enhancing properties. Plants demonstrate great versatility for the treatment of a broad variety of health needs. Plants can cleanse the bowels, open congested sinuses, help mend broken bones, stimulate the brain, ease pain, aid digestion, and have a thousand other purposes. Topically, plants can repair damaged skin, soothe a wound, improve complexion, heal bruises, and relieve aching muscles. Plant medicines overall are far safer, gentler, and better for human health than synthetic drugs. Nature offers plants that interact with every system in the body and every conceivable human function, from respiration to circulation, from nerve function to digestion, and for sexual enhancement.

For at least a few thousand years, humans have employed various plants in a variety of ways to perk up libido, to produce harder erections and more copious lubrication, and to generate more ecstatic sexual satisfaction. Accounts of their effects have passed from one generation to another, and from one land to the next. *Keep in mind that people have no reasonable motive to pass on misinformation about the effects of a plant for a long time. Instead, people pass on useful information that can be employed to the advantage of others.* Virtually every culture has its prized sexual plant secret. Some work better than others, and a handful work very well indeed. When it comes to sex, satisfaction is the name of the game. People use these hot plants because they produce the desired results.

This book is not intended to cure any serious sexual problem. If you suffer from erectile dysfunction, for example, the cause may be cardiovascular disease. Or, the cause may be neurological. Or diabetes. It is wise to consult a physician to rule out any serious chronic disease. On the other hand, erectile dysfunction, loss of libido, or reduced sexual pleasure may result from the forces of stress, poor diet, or general fatigue. With chronic disease factors ruled out, the hot plants may help to restore you to full sexual vitality.

The hot plants work by various means. Some boost testosterone, which enhances libido in both men and women. Some improve circulation in fine vessels, thereby enhancing erectile function. Some work by eliminating deleterious chemicals produced in the body by stress that impair sexual function in a variety of insidious ways. Some boost the production of neu-rotransmitters in the brain that directly affect sexual desire and function. Perhaps you just want to take your sexual experi-ence up a notch, build a hotter fire, stoke the flames of passion. The hot plants will help you to do that. They are, in fact, very fine agents for enhancing an already healthy sexual experience. They make sex a bit more urgent, sensitivity more acute, or-gasm more like Chinese New Year fireworks. The hot plants are sexual allies. They will make you hotter, harder, more sexually hungry and alive. They will push you to new heights of plea-sure and make your juices flow more strongly.

So come with me on this exploration of nature's agents of desire, from country to country and continent to continent. I promise you, there is sexual adventure in the hot plants.

THE OLDEST FOREST

Tongkat Ali

IN DENSELY SHADED GREENERY ON A STEEP HILL IN THE OLD-est rain forest in the world, I stood soaking wet from a mad downpour. Before me, three Orang Asli—Malaysia's aboriginal people—chopped a mature Tongkat Ali root, one of the most powerful aphrodisiac plants on earth, out of dense soil on a dangerous slope. I kept a watchful eye for deadly snakes: red-headed kraits and king cobras in particular. That morning, one of our party had spotted two adult tigers crossing a road. Re-searching sex-enhancing plants often puts me in remote places with indigenous people who know the harvesting, preparation, and uses of the native botanical pharmacopoeia. In this in-stance, the trail led me to Malaysia to research Tongkat Ali.

Tongkat Ali is a popular folk name for *Eurycoma longifolia*, a medium-size slender tree reaching ten meters in height. The name Tongkat Ali means "Ali's walking stick." Another folk name for the plant is Longjack. By any moniker, Tongkat Ali is native to Malaysia, lower Burma, Thailand, and Indonesia. The plant thrives in shade and flourishes under the canopy of the rain forest. The root is employed as a traditional remedy for the treatment of malaria, high blood pressure, fevers, fatigue, loss of sexual desire, and impotence. Tongkat Ali enjoys a long history of traditional use and a growing body of serious science corroborating its effectiveness. The plant is a natural wonder. In Malaysia, Tongkat Ali is a national treasure and the object of a sexual potency craze. It is also an ingredient found in more than three hundred products, from root chips to herbal syrups, capsules, and popular soft drinks. Southeast Asian men and women enjoy Tongkat Ali in a plethora of forms, for its sex-enhancing properties.

Nobody knows how long Tongkat Ali has been employed for medicinal purposes, but its documented use dates back to the 1700s. My journey to the Malaysian peninsula was inspired by Annie Eng, who first briefed me about the plant at a natural products convention a few years ago. Annie grew up in Penang state in Malaysia, and eventually moved to Chicago to study business and finance. She worked as a successful stock broker for years, but Malaysia's most famous plant, Tongkat Ali, stuck in her mind. She made connections with scientists and processors in Malaysia, started a company called Herbal Powers, and began to sell a concentrated extract of Tongkat Ali called LJ100 in the U.S. market. And she persistently chased down anybody who she sensed might advance her cause.

Annie gave me samples of Tongkat Ali to try. She called. She sent e-mails. She mailed me studies. Over time, I paid increasingly close attention, gave keen consideration to what she had sent me, and realized that she was onto something very big. After more than a year and a half of conversations, after swallowing innumerable samples, and reading studies and any available literature on Tongkat Ali, I found myself on a jet with Annie Eng, heading toward the Malaysian capital of Kuala Lumpur.

With the Original People

In Malaysia we traveled with an entourage of at least ten, including scientific and business contacts associated with Annie, and a television production crew called Taiping Broadcasting. We had arranged to shoot the entire research trip as a documentary to air on Malaysian television. I was the on-air protagonist, a medicine hunter on the trail of one of nature's most potent sex-enhancing herbs. Our group moved about in a Land Cruiser, a pickup truck and van combined, making our way from city to country. We packed a small mountain of photographic, video and sound equipment, drinking water, clothing, and personal effects.

The trail led us up north in Perak state near the town of Gerik to an Orang Asli village. The original inhabitants of peninsular Malaysia, today about 80,000 Orang Asli remain scattered throughout the country. Though many have moved to cities and towns, have married non-aboriginals, and have been assimilated into modern culture, a number of Orang Asli choose to live in settlements and villages in the forest, leading simpler lives absent of most modern amenities. The Orang Asli are intimately familiar with the Malaysian rain forest. They know the plants, the animals, the weather, and the various skills required to survive and thrive in the dense jungle. Thanks to arrangements made by Malaysian medicinal plant expert Dr. Azrae Idris, we were scheduled to meet with a group of Orang Alsi who had agreed to guide us into the forest, to find a mature Tongkat Ali tree, and to harvest the root. Our aim was to see and film the traditional way that Tongkat Ali is harvested in the wild.

Once our convoy arrived at the village, we met the village

head man, Haliban. At Haliban's direction we would travel into the forest to harvest Tongkat Ali. One of our crew, Nazar, dispensed candy to a giggling and excited throng of Orang Asli children. We spent an hour or so videotaping and shooting photographs of the village people and our crew. Our visit was a big event for them, with our cameras and microphones and gear, and meeting the Orang Asli people were an equally big event for us. They were our much-needed guides and allies in unfamiliar terrain. After a time, Haliban gave an approving nod, then along with five other native men led us into the woods.

Hiking into the oldest rain forest in the world proved breathtakingly beautiful, if challenging. A roasting equatorial sun kept the temperature hovering in the mid 30s C (high 90s F). Humidity hung in the air like a wet towel at about 98 percent, so we were drenched with streaming sweat from the very onset of our hike. As we moved into the steep hills of the forest with the Orang Asli in the lead, tripper vines by the hundreds wrapped around our ankles and impeded our progress. We remained vigilant for poisonous snakes, though they'd be almost impossible to spot in the dense undergrowth. The Malaysian rain forest is home to over twenty species of highly poisonous snakes, including a few that are are deadly and aggressive, like the Russell's viper and the king cobra. We also kept a sharp lookout for toxic giant centipedes, fist-size black scorpions, fire ants, and sharp bamboo. What looked like useful handholds often bore sharp spines and spikes. Many vines and small trees were attached to nothing, so we had to test each one before hanging on and hoisting ourselves up slippery inclines. The forest is home to wild elephants, tigers, and the occasional black leopard, but we were not fortunate enough to catch even a glimpse of those beautiful and elusive animals.

Despite the slow and arduous hike, the rain forest proved to be a spectacle of natural beauty, featuring the greatest diversity of plant life of any forest on earth. The smells were rich: the greenery of the forest, along with decomposing plant material on the forest floor, created complex aromas, ranging from floral to fecal. As we walked along we encountered thousands of dragonflies and heard the calls of many birds. Along the way we stopped to admire giant wild ginger and exotic blossoms. We heard monkeys making a cacophonous racket faraway.

After a full morning of hiking we came upon a small Tongkat Ali tree. Dr. Azrae, who knows a great deal about the growth of Tongkat Ali, figured that the little tree was about three years old, and therefore unsuitable for our purposes. A Tongkat Ali tree needs to be at least five years old before it is ready for harvesting, so we moved on. Soon after, Dr. Azrae spotted, on a very steep hillside, a Tongkat Ali tree with a trunk about five inches in diameter, which he estimated to be at least fifteen years old. It was a perfect specimen to harvest and would yield a root of at least ten kilos in weight. Our practical problem would be to arrange ourselves and the video camera to avoid tumbling down the sharp and dangerous incline into a ravine of snakes, thorns, and razor bamboo.

To clear some of the foliage from above the Tongkat Ali tree, an Orang Asli named Din removed his sneakers and scampered up the slender trunk as easily as if it were a flight of stairs. He climbed to a height of about twenty feet, balancing himself with one foot on the Tongkat Ali tree and the other on another tree. With both trees swaying back and forth, he worked with a machete, hacking away at overhead branches as easily as if he were working on flat, level ground. For most modern people, climbing a tree in such a manner would be completely out of the question but to some of the Orang Asli, climbing trees with such agility is a natural ability acquired and mastered early in life. Many indigenous native people possess extraordinary natural skills and can survive and thrive in environments in which more modernized people would perish.

Before we could get set up, we heard the sound of rain moving toward us very quickly. The shower hit overhead, and the downpour became intense. Soon we were soaked through our underwear and socks. The rain felt marvelously refreshing, and I was disappointed when it stopped only ten minutes after it began.

Once the branches overhead were cleared, three of the Orang Asli began harvesting the Tongkat Ali root. Using only a small pick and a chopping blade, the men dug away soil from around the base of the Tongkat Ali tree. The root was as big around as a man's leg and about four feet long. This made for hard labor in the sweltering forest. The Orang Asli typically earn about $4 Ringhitt (3.8 RM equals about a $1.50 U.S.) per kilo of root for their labor. And keep in mind, they have to hike out of the forest, and carry the freshly harvested Tongkat Ali root with them. And yet, the activity is profitable for them, and they harvest Tongkat Ali to garner cash for clothing and other goods.

The difficulty of harvesting Tongkat Ali in the wild is one very good reason to cultivate the trees in plantations, but there's a more important reason to cultivate Tongkat Ali. As this traditional plant remedy becomes more popular, supplies of Tongkat Ali in the wild will inevitably decrease. Over time, this tree could become endangered. To preserve the natural environment and to protect remaining wild specimens of Tongkat Ali, Malaysia will need to establish large plantations of this tree. At present, the country's largest oil palm producer, Golden Hope, is establishing a ten thousand acre plantation of Tongkat Ali. Smaller plantations are also in process of starting up, but many more will be needed. In order to ensure a consistent supply of Tongkat Ali for the future, hundreds of thousands of acres will need to be dedicated to its cultivation. The Malaysian government is enthusiastic about the future of Tongkat Ali and is already providing economic support for its development.

The Testosterone Builder

Tongkat Ali is more than just a pretty name. It is a scientifically studied plant whose powers hold up brilliantly under close scrutiny. The root contains a plethora of beneficial compounds, including potent protective antioxidants that inhibit cellular aging. Other phytochemicals in Tongkat Ali are antiviral, anti-malarial, and anticarcinogenic. Still others combat high blood pressure and quell dysentery. Compound called quassinoids in the root prove twice as potent as aspirin against fevers. The root is a natural medicine chest, suitable for broad use. A scientific collaboration between Malaysian researchers and drug chemists in the United States has identified significant anti-cancer activity in Tongkat Ali, presumably due to certain quassinoids and alkaloids. The root's powerful antiviral compounds are the subjects of ongoing close investigation and drug development as well.

Even with its other medical applications, what excites most people about Tongkat Ali is that the root significantly boosts sex drive and function in men and women, by increasing testosterone. Agents identified as glycoproteins are believed to be the sex-promoting ingredients in the plant. This discovery, the result of years of painstaking research, is the work of Dr. Johari Saad, who is known as the "King of Tongkat Ali." A brilliant scientist, inventor, engineer, and former professor at the University of Malaysia, Dr. Johari, or Joe, as he is called, has conducted the definitive animal research on Tongkat Ali and developed a novel and proprietary method of extracting the beneficial compounds from the root. Joe and I spent many long hours discussing Tongkat Ali and other Malaysian medicinal plants as our convoy made its way on the medicine trail.

"In our studies, we looked at what was happening with animals when we gave them a water soluble extract of Tongkat Ali," Joe explained to me. "It basically came down to four categories: increased testosterone; increased energy; inhibition of SHBG, which is sex hormone binding globulin; and increased muscle mass." His four discoveries are highly significant and have greatly advanced knowledge of the biological effects of this extraordinary plant.

When given Tongkat Ali extract, animals copulate three to four times more frequently than normal. This is due, as it turns out, to a significant increase in testosterone. In fact, testosterone levels in animals given Tongkat Ali increase an unprecedented three to four times on average. This is an astounding increase in the sex hormone most closely associated with libido. Though animal results do not always guarantee identical activity in people, I later discovered that the same testosterone-boosting effect does occur in human studies. In laboratory tests on human testicular tissue, Tongkat Ali extract increased the formation of testosterone fourfold.

Increasing testosterone is the key factor in increasing sex drive. Testosterone is the most important of the male sex hormones, known as androgens, produced in the gonads. Testosterone plays a key role in the development and maturity of male sex organs. The hormone promotes secondary sex characteristics including the appearance of facial hair, enlargement of the larynx (producing a deeper voice), sexual desire, and sexual behavior. Testosterone also stimulates metabolism, promotes lypolisis (burning of fat), increases the formation of red blood cells, and accelerates muscle growth. But testosterone is not just a sex booster for men. Women also produce testosterone, about 5 to 10 percent the amount produced in men. In women, this vital hormone also stimulates sex drive.

There is a problem relative to testosterone, and Tongkat Ali offers a solution. From age thirty or so, blood levels of the hormone decline at a rate of about 2 percent per year. By age forty-five, a man may have only 60 percent of the testosterone he had at age twenty-five. By age fifty, the level is around 55 percent. The level will vary from one person to another. A man who exercises is likely to keep a somewhat higher level of testosterone. Those who smoke or drink heavily will lose more of this hormone more quickly. As testosterone decreases in the body, muscle tone, energy, and sex drive all begin to decline. The same decline in testosterone occurs in women, though the amounts of testosterone involved are lower than in men. In both sexes, sex drive, sexual function, rate of fat metabolism, and energy decline into middle age.

What if you could boost your testosterone levels to more youthful levels? With Tongkat Ali extract you can. And that makes Tongkat Ali a sexual fountain of youth. Dr. Johari also found that Tongkat Ali extract inhibits sex hormone binding globulin. By inhibiting this agent, more free testosterone remains in the blood. This additional testosterone slows the aging process, improving energy and sexual function, helping to reduce body fat, and reducing risk factors associated with cardiovascular disease. Consuming a properly made extract of the plant increases testosterone significantly in both animals and humans.

What About Women?

If you stick with me through this book, you will learn a lot about natural botanical aphrodisiacs. There are fewer sexual studies with women than with men. The reason for this is a systemic bias that runs across cultures and continents. I once read that if men menstruated, there would be a U.S. Department of Dysmenorrhea. Men tend to run countries, governments, and economies, they care a great deal more about male sexual issues and needs than those of women. A number of studies on men show that various hot plants work to build libido and to improve sexual function. But comparable studies on women do not exist. With Tongkat Ali, for example, clinical studies of men demonstrates what this plant does and why. To make the same case for women, we must examine two factors: mechanism of action and long-term cultural use.

In terms of mechanism of action, Tongkat Ali works in the body as a testosterone builder. In women as in men, testosterone is extremely important to sexual function and pleasure. This powerful hormone is the key to a proactive sex drive in women. Testosterone is not only a trigger of women's libido, it is also essential to pleasure. Testosterone produces erotic sensitivity of the clitoris, breasts, and nipples. Testosterone flips the pleasure switches on women's erogenous zones. Testosterone also acts in women as an antidepressant and confidence-boosting agent. Though women produce far less testosterone than men, it is the active agent for their sex drive. Testosterone levels decline in women after age thirty as they do in men, which is why Tongkat Ali can provide a major boost to a woman's sexual desire and pleasure.

This brings us to long-term cultural use. Women have employed Tongkat Ali as an aphrodisiac, for centuries at least. They do so because Tongkat Ali works. Those of us who work in the field of ethnobotany understand that there is simply no incentive whatsoever for a large population of people to use a plant for a particular purpose over many generations if that plant does not deliver. Indigenous people have long ago figured out what plants work for what health needs. Science may help to corroborate the use of traditional plant remedies, and scientific investigation often leads to an explanation of how plants work in the body, but scientific studies do not "validate" long-term plant use. Plant use is valid as determined by extensive human experience. Women have long gotten powerful sexual benefits from Tongkat Ali. This is an equal opportunity hot plant of the highest possible order.

In both men and women, pharmaceutical testosterone has been successfully used as a therapeutic aid in cases of low sex drive. The hormone has also been used to treat some cases of erectile dysfunction in men. With Tongkat Ali, we have a safe, natural plant agent that causes the body to produce its own testosterone, boosting sexual desire and function. Tongkat Ali gets to the aboslute essence of human sex drive and improves it.

And Boom Again

Tongkat Ali extract also greatly increases ATP production. ATP, or adenosine triphosphate, is the basic unit of energy in the body, responsible for keeping us alive and going. By increasing ATP, overall energy and vitality are increased. Most people want more energy, and Tongkat Ali provides it, without hyperstimulation, jittery nerves, or insomnia. Promoting human energy production is a valuable enough health benefit by itself to make Tongkat Ali an enduring superstar of medicinal plants. Energy is a functional attribute likely desired and prized more than any other.

Seiful, one of the all-time greatest field hockey players in Malaysia and a national hero, swears by Tongkat Ali. At age thirty-eight, Seiful is past his athletic prime, but is still a highly distinguished player. The former captain of Malaysia's national field hockey team has played in three Olympics and in one World Cup. He remains one of the hardest hitters in all of Malaysia, and is an active player today. Seiful attributes his remarkable energy and stamina in part to the Tongkat Ali extract developed by Dr. Johari. "The Tongkat Ali definitely helps me. I find it gives me much more energy," he told me before a game. Did Seiful recommend the plant to his friends? He smiled. "Yes, I have told a lot of players. They use Tongkat Ali, and it helps them. Many hockey players use Tongkat Ali now." As athletes in other parts of the world experience the benefits of Tongkat Ali, the extract will most likely become part of every serious training regime.

Athletes and bodybuilders will buy any agent that boosts performance or muscle mass. Endocrinologists have known for a long time that testosterone increases the body's ratio of lean muscle mass to fat. In both animals and humans, Tongkat Ali extract increases muscle mass. In a study of men, half of the subjects ingested Tongkat Ali extract and half did not. In an eight-week physical training program, the men who consumed

Tongkat Ali extract experienced greater gains in muscle mass and strength than those who did not. This demonstrates the powerful anabolic properties of Tongkat Ali. Thanks to this significant discovery, a growing number of athletes and body-builders now use Tongkat Ali extract as an androgen to improve muscle size and strength and to enhance sports performance. Tongkat Ali is the testosterone-boosting, muscle-enhancing titan of the plant kingdom. Instead of turning to the use of dangerous and potentially lethal steroids, perhaps more athletes will opt for Tongkat Ali.

The Extract Secret

"One of the things we found is that when organic solvents are used to extract Tongkat Ali, you get a number of toxic compounds, especially the quassinoids, in the extract. So I had to come up with an extract that would be safe and effective," Dr. Johari explained. Developing a good method of extraction can be very difficult. To do so, Dr. Johari not only needed to devise a method but had to engineer and build a state-of-the-art extraction facility, capable of large-scale production.

Joe explained that "the use of alcohol or other organic extraction solvents, such as hexane or acetone, produces an extract with an unacceptable level of toxic compounds. Interestingly, these compounds are also medicinally beneficial—for fighting some types of cancers and viruses. But for everyday use, they should only be consumed in microscopic amounts." When I asked him how much Tongkat Ali extract people should take, he said, "We have found that men need about 100 mg (milligrams) of extract per day, while women need about 50 mg."

With this in mind, Dr. Johari began to experiment with a

water extract. Using water, pressure, a very specific range of temperature, and a precise amount of time, Joe was able to develop a proprietary Tongkat Ali extract with a very low quassinoid level, but with high amounts of the active glycoproteins. That extract has been used in all the animal and human studies that have been conducted on Tongkat Ali. In the United States Dr. Johari's proprietary Tongkat Ali extract goes by the name LJ100.

The best botanical companies in the world engage in this kind of activity, developing a proprietary manufacturing method for a plant extract, and then conducting animal and human trials to verify the efficacy of the product. In this way legitimate companies can separate themselves from the vast range of imitators, wannabes, fakers, and fly-by-night outfits who do not even know how to spell the word *science,* let alone conduct any. In any product category, from toasters to computers to canned soups, there are fine quality products and others that aren't worth using. In this book, I do my best to identify those companies and extracts that exemplify proper development and testing, sorting out the good products from the junk.

The Woman Herbalist

About two hours north of Kuala Lumpur, we pulled up to a traditional Malay house in the countryside outside the town of Ipoh. On stilts and surrounded by flower gardens, the picturesque house was one of increasingly rare design. With its peaked roof and weathered shingles, the house stood as a reminder of days past. By arrangement through Dr. Azrae, we were there to meet with Kak Yang, a traditional woman herbalist, or *bomoh.* On arriving, we were greeted by her family of six. They had been busy setting up all the necessary elements for making a traditional herbal formula, or *jamu.* After we shook hands all around, we were led to a blanket-sized woven rattan mat on the ground, covered with numerous medicinal herbs and several implements used in their preparation.

Kak Yang appeared dressed in splendid silks as if she were attending an imperial ball. Her ample breasts strained at the buttons of a tight, brocaded vest adorned with intricate dragon designs in gold and silver thread. Tall and big boned, Kak Yang carried herself like an individual assured of success, bearing a confidence that often accompanies knowledge. She explained that she worked with many people in the area and had helped many with their health problems. I asked how she got started learning about medicinal herbs. "My mother," she told me. "My great-great-grandmother was an herbalist, and then my great-grandmother, and my grandmother, and my mother. I am the fifth generation of women in my family who practice traditional herbal medicine. Ever since I was a little girl, I helped my mother when she would prepare remedies. I helped her to pick plants as well, and she taught me all about preparing them and using them." As I find in so many cultures, women are the primary keepers of herbal wisdom. Even when I ask male herbalists in other countries where they learned their craft, most say their mother or grandmother.

I wanted to see the traditional preparation of a *jamu,* with Tongkat Ali as the primary ingredient. Kak Yang was ready with at least a dozen herbal ingredients piled onto a wide rattan tray. I recognized Tongkat Ali, cinnamon bark, dried ginger root, and dried turmeric root. As the cameras rolled, Kak Yang first roasted the large pile of dried herbs in a black iron wok over an open fire. "This will make the herbs easier to pound into powder," she explained. "It dries them more, and they will be brittle. So they will break apart with less work." After the roasting process was completed, Kak Yang emptied the herbs into a deep wooden pounding vessel. Hefting a heavy rod of iron, she beat the herb chunks in the vessel with the rod end, breaking them up into increasingly smaller pieces as she labored in the hot sun. She had large, strong hands. Sweat droplets sprouted on Kak Yang's brow, but she didn't get even a speck of dust on her beautiful silks.

After about twenty minutes of pounding, Kak Yang had reduced much of the herbal pile to dust. She dumped the pounded herbs onto a fine sifter and shook it over a spread piece of newspaper. The fine powder that made it through the mesh was the *jamu,* the formula. "Now you can use this *jamu* in this form, or you can make it into what we call *majoon,* by adding honey and rolling it into balls. Or you can also cook it in oil and make a massage preparation." I put a pinch of the formula in my mouth. It was quite bitter, mostly due to the Tongkat Ali, which made up about half of the mix. I asked if she would tell me about her experiences with Tongkat Ali for both men and women. "I make formulas for men and women with Tongkat Ali, and it is very good to increase sexual vitality in either case. I have been making Tongkat Ali *jamu* for several years now, and I put it into capsules, and sell the products for men and women in my little store in Ipoh. These products have become quite famous in this area, because they make men and women very sexual." Does Tongkat Ali help men or women to regain sexual function? "Sometimes they come to me and they aren't interested in sex, or men can't get erect. After taking one of my Tongkat Ali formulas for more than twenty-four days, they usually improve greatly."

Kak Yang was describing the way that traditional herbal healers have worked throughout human history. People seek the counsel of wise herbalists, who have learned about the medicinal uses of plants and have helped others with myriad health problems. The education of the traditional plant healer does not take place in classrooms and labs, but becoming an expert traditional healer requires no less diligent study, no less attention to detail and knowledge of broad and interconnected disciplines. The traditional healer must know how to diagnose correctly health disorders of all kinds. They are, as a rule, general practitioners, and must be able to help knit a broken bone as well as stop diarrhea, get rid of a persistent cough, or help to relieve headaches. He or she must also know the endemic plants of their region, when and how to harvest them, what parts to use, how to prepare them, and how and when to administer remedies made from them. Traditional healers know how to make teas and extracts, potions and preparations of all kinds, from syrups and pastes to ointments and pessaries.

Kak Yang proudly showed us a number of her own bottled, labeled products, which contained encapsulated formulas based primarily around Tongkat Ali. Each product bore a proud photo of a smiling, elegantly dressed Kak Yang on the label as a sign of authenticity. She was pleased by the positive market reception to her products. She was also generous and gave a free bottle of Tongkat Ali *jamu* capsules to everyone in our crew. As we were packing up to leave, Kak Yang beckoned me aside and discreetly revealed a small bottle of dark oil. She leaned in close and pressed the bottle into my hand. "This is for your penis. If you like it, call me and tell me your experience." I thanked her, expressing appreciation for the gift and for her company. All of us shook hands all around. As we drove off I wondered to myself exactly what I was supposed to do with the oil.

The Sex Doctor

Back in the capital of Kuala Lumpur, the crew and I temporarily disrupted the peace at the Human Reproduction Specialist Centre. We had a scheduled meeting with Dr. Ismail Tambi, a medical doctor who specializes in the study and treatment of reproductive disorders of all kinds. When we arrived, the four women behind the reception desk spoke excitedly about our video shoot. Our arrival was apparently the most stimulating local event in quite some time. We shot video footage of the receptionists, much to their delight.

Dr. Ismail Tambi turned out to be gracious and articulate, looking very much the impeccable physician in a trim white coat. Dr. Tambi is one of the foremost experts on reproductive health in Southeast Asia. He works with men and women in all cases of sexual dysfunction, reproductive disorders, and fertility problems. He is also the leading medical expert on the effects of Tongkat Ali root extract on human subjects. In his work with men, Dr. Tambi has found that use of Tongkat Ali extract significantly increases testosterone production. "I was very skeptical at first about this type of thing, using some plant to change hormone levels. But I did some work with it, and Tongkat Ali turned out to be highly potent. In our studies, we found that Tongkat Ali extract increased the serum level of testosterone considerably." I asked Dr. Tambi if the men in his study experienced renewed sexual vitality or heightened sexual

desire. "Oh, yes, most definitely. The men found that Tongkat
Ali boosted their sex drive quite a lot. I think that for low libido, Tongkat Ali extract is very valuable. I have seen this result
for myself and can say that this plant really works." This finding confirms traditional use of Tongkat Ali for the enhancement of libido. I asked Dr. Tambi if the same would apply to
women, who secrete only about 5 to 10 percent as much
testosterone as men. "Yes, it certainly should boost libido in
women as well, as testosterone is essential to a woman's sexual
desire. Women have used Tongkat Ali for a very long time in
this culture," he added.

Dr. Tambi conducted the PADAM study, in which he investigated partial androgen deficiency in males. He selected thirty
adult males of various ages, assessed their testosterone levels,
and then gave them 100 mg of Tongkat Ali extract daily. The
testosterone levels of all the subjects rose, from somewhat to a
lot, depending on age. Dr Tambi's study resulted in a 91 percent improvement in libido, a reported 73 percent improvement in sexual function, and an 82 percent psychological
improvement relative to sex among the men who participated
in the study. His work shows that while the level of testosterone in the blood decreases with age, Tongkat Ali can reele-
vate the level of this important sex hormone.

A Tongkat Ali Blizzard

The Chow Kit Market is one of the busiest markets in
Malaysia's capital of Kuala Lumpur. Chow Kit features numerous stalls where fresh and dried herbs are sold. Some of the
herbs, like ginger and turmeric, are for cooking. Some of the

herbs are used primarily for medicinal purposes, for a broad range of health needs. People go to Chow Kit to buy medicinal plants for common health needs: relieving an upset stomach, treating a headache, enhancing sexual function, promoting a good night's sleep. In Chow Kit, shops and stalls of all sizes sell a huge selection of Tongkat Ali products, from whole and chopped root to capsules and beverages. Traditional *jamu* formulas containing Tongkat Ali are also common there. At Chow Kit, I cruised the market with Dr. Johari, stopping at small herbal stalls to examine the many Tongkat Ali products on display.

In one stall we spoke with a glassy-eyed, very excited proprietor named Osman. "Why do you have so many Tongkat Ali products?" I asked.

Osman lit up as though I had bonked him on the head. "Sex, for sex. Mostly sex." He pointed to labels featuring muscled men, men and women embracing, hearts, and various other graphics connoting raw animal power, togetherness, or love.

"Are these products very popular?" I pointed to Tongkat Ali coffee mix, Tongkat Ali fruit drinks, syrups, bags of root chips, bottles of capsules.

Osman grinned hard. "Oh yes, very popular. So popular you cannot imagine. All of them. Very, very popular. Men and women all buy them, every day." Osman turned out to be the most enthusiastic of the shopkeepers with whom we spoke in Chow Kit, but answers to similar questions were consistent. Tongkat Ali, in virtually any and all forms, was a booming product category, with high demand. Virtually every stall in the market featured a prominent display of Tongkat Ali products catering to men and women.

A Tongkat Ali Garden

Our caravan made its way to FRIM, the Forestry Research Institute of Malaysia. As part of its commitment to the future of Tongkat Ali, the Malaysian government is investigating the cultivation of this valuable medicinal plant. Occupying more than three thousand lush green acres, FRIM runs a small experimental Tongkat Ali plot at the Kepong Botanical Garden in Kuala Lumpur. Agricultural researchers are using that plot and others to determine the best growing conditions for Tongkat Ali. Azrae, Joe, Annie, and I threaded our way around bushes and bamboo to reach the plot. There, several dozen young Tongkat Ali trees grew in rows.

Joe commented on the agricultural research being conducted on Tongkat Ali. "Every six months, researchers pull around twenty of these trees, to assess root size and weight. This research will help Tongkat Ali to make the transition from a wild forest plant to a plantation crop. But I can see here that the trees need more shade. They like shade, not direct sun. Still, it's good that the government is taking an active interest in Tongkat Ali." One thing was clear to me, that while the actual growing methods in the FRIM garden may need to be tweaked, the Malaysian government recognizes a future agricultural crop in Tongkat Ali.

A Tea Break

We were near the end of our project. We had covered many hundreds of kilometers of territory, shot hour upon hour of video footage, and had interviewed many experts about Tongkat Ali. We were tired and ready to stop living out of suitcases. At the very least, we were due for a good tea break. A tea break in the middle of the day is an old and very welcome tradition. We headed into a small shop on a dusty road on the outskirts of Kuala Lumpur, for *the tarik* (pronounced *tay tareek*), or "pulled" tea. The tea is called pulled, because it is poured through the air a couple of feet from one pot to another, to mix and cool it. *The tarik* Tongkat Ali made with is a popular beverage today as in times past. But now, the Tongkat Ali tea is usually made from a pre-mix somewhat like instant coffee, instead of by the labor-intensive method of chopping, boiling, and straining the roots.

Annie, Azrae, Joe, and I sat under a fan, which whooshed around 36° C (100° F) hot air. A long lean waiter was preparing *the tarik* for us. The modern Tongkat Ali *the tarik* tasted great, offering delicious refreshment, and a comfortable escape from the hot midday sun. Drinking our Tongkat Ali tea, we recapped all that we had seen and done.

We had known prior to coming together that Tongkat Ali is a special plant. But even for seasoned veterans like Azrae and Joe, our trip had further affirmed that Tongkat Ali is a rare health treasure. This plant has been used as a traditional remedy for centuries. And yet today, Tongkat Ali is entering a whole new era of use. Thanks to dedicated scientists, modern manufacturing, governmental support, and consumer demand, Tongkat Ali has been transformed into a modern health product.

Tongkat Ali is on the move, from the borders of Malaysia to ports of call around the globe. The plant is becoming popular in the Middle East, in Japan, and in the United States. Articles and TV programs extol the virtues of Tongkat Ali. A blizzard of Tongkat Ali products have hit the market and the plant is now ready for its time in the international health spotlight. Tongkat Ali is hot indeed, one of the greatest of all the aphrodisiac plants. This ancient remedy from the oldest rain forest on earth is now about to meet the sexual needs of millions of people worldwide.

Using Tongkat Ali

Dr. Johari, Dr. Tambi, and other experts involved with this plant recommend around 100 milligrams of concentrated, water-extracted Tongkat Ali daily for men and around 50 milligrams for women, standardized to approximately 22 percent glycoproteins. In the resources section at the end of this book, you will find my recommendations for high-quality brands of Tongkat Ali.

FROM RUSSIA WITH LOVE

Rhodiola rosea

STRESS CAN MAKE A MESS OF YOUR LOVE LIFE IN INSIDIOUS ways. In fact, stress causes innumerable flaccid erections, dry vaginas, and cases of lost sexual desire in men and women. Physical, emotional, and mental stress can be caused by many circumstances. Overly cramped schedules, too many responsibilities, not enough fun, poor nutrition, long commutes, work pressures, sickness, financial struggles, and a thousand other matters can drive us to the edge and undermine our well-being, reducing our energy and joy and dampening desire.

Stress isn't just in the head. Its effects contribute to cardiovascular disease, nervous disorders, poor digestive function, compromised immunity, chronic fatigue, depression, and sleeplessness. Left unchecked, stress causes biochemical damage that results in reduced sexual desire and impaired sexual function in men and women. Stress has no gender bias—it is an equal opportunity antagonist. The science of psychoneuroimmunology has discovered that a cascade of chemical events triggered by stress causes a host of health problems such as those above, and becomes self-reinforcing. The more stress we endure, the more self-perpetuating becomes our response to stress, until it is all so ratcheted up we function poorly. Even when the stress factors are removed, the damage is done. Stress blows an ill wind through the bedroom.

Bound For Siberia

You could say that stress put me on the road to Siberia. More accurately, you could say that the search for an antistress agent of superior power, possessed of extraordinary reinvigorating properties, sent me to that vast and mysterious land. I will travel just about anywhere to find a cure. Since Siberia was the place to find a cure for stress-induced systemic and sexual devastation, I was on my way.

In Siberia I intended to research a plant that is known to reverse the ravages of stress, restore healthy physical and mental function, rekindle passion, and renew loving ability in both men and women. That plant, *Rhodiola rosea,* was the object of my desire. I had read about *Rhodiola rosea* for years. Medicinal uses of the plant were first noted by the Greek physician Dioscorides, around 77 B.C. From that time on, the plant gained a reputation for its extraordinary healing properties. The botanist Linnaeus named it *Rhodiola rosea,* in reference to the roselike aroma of the root. He also ascribed numerous healing properties to the root, including uses for headache and hysteria. The plant has long been part of the traditional medicines of Russia and Scandinavia, and since the early 1700s, hundreds of preparations made from *Rhodiola rosea* have been marketed. The plant is most commonly referred to simply as Rhodiola, but this confuses the issue somewhat, as there are many species of Rhodiola. *Rhodiola rosea* specifically has been studied extensively: it is a proven miracle of nature and an effective hot plant.

In traditional folk medicine, *Rhodiola rosea* has been employed to promote energy and stamina, to banish fatigue, to restore the nervous system after exhaustion, to boost sexual desire, and to treat impotence. In antiquity, preparations of the root were used to treat colds, flu, depression, cancer, and gastrointestinal complaints. Methods of preparation and locations of plants were often jealously guarded by families of healers and *Rhodiola rosea* became such a legendary invigorating agent and booster of sexual potency that Chinese emperors sent expeditions to Siberia expressly to gather the root.

In the 1990s, a few supplement makers put out *Rhodiola rosea* products in the United States, but they were poorly marketed and never made much of a splash. Nonetheless, as I dug into existing research on the herb, I was sure that it was one of the great hot plants. As a faculty member in the Medicinal Plant Program at the University of Massachusetts at Amherst, I am accustomed to researching existing science on any particular plant. As the university's explorer in residence, I am keen to jump on a jet and head off to research any botanical that may benefit humanity. I made some reliable contacts in Central Siberia, packed my luggage, and headed out with notebook and camera, a bag full of film, and the inspiring promise of discovery that so often characterizes my trips.

Siberia represents a little-tapped frontier of botanical riches. I intended to gain as much understanding as possible of the range and scope of what could be found there, while specifically investigating *Rhodiola rosea*. I made plans to meet with botanical experts, plant chemists, traditional healers, herbal traders, and herb hunters and gatherers. I also hoped to garner information on the extent of current cultural use of Siberian medicinal botanicals.

Comprising the entire upper third of Asia, the vast region of Siberia stretches from the Ural Mountains in the west to the Pacific Ocean in the east. Covering 2,900,000 square miles, Siberia's area is a full 80 percent of that of the United States, with regional diversity ranging from scenic mountains to tundra with bogs so deep they can swallow a person whole. The area I was headed to, central Siberia, is home to the Altay, a 100,000-square-mile region of mountains, rushing rivers, and more than 3,000 lakes, bordering both Mongolia and Kazahkstan. The Altay is also one of the primary collection areas for *Rhodiola rosea*, also known as golden root. A well-studied adaptogen, Rhodiola defends the body overall and protects general health and well-being. Its anti-stress and fatigue-fighting properties make it one of the most popular botanicals in all of Siberia. And its promotion of energy, endurance, and stamina makes *Rhodiola rosea* a valuable aid for athletes. Extracts from the roots of the plant have been used by Eastern Bloc athletes for decades to improve overall performance. The root has also enjoyed a very long history for promoting sexual vigor and prowess.

My air travel route took me from Boston to London to the great Russian capital, Moscow. From there I boarded a giant Aeroflot IL86, a sort of immense bus with wings, and shuddered off into blue Russian skies on the five-hour flight to Novosibirsk. Once in Siberia's largest city, I met my hosts and guides, herbal traders Marat Khamzin and Vadim Kolpakov of Russian Natural Products. Ideal advisers and companions on the medicine trail, they export Siberian botanicals to other countries, own an impressive herbal tea business, operate seven pharmacies that feature Siberian botanical remedies, and are connected with herbal traders all over Siberia. Marat and Vadim proved unfailingly helpful and generous as we made our way.

What the Experts Say

The area of Novosibirsk is home to the Central Siberian Botanical Garden. Funded by the Russian government, the ten-thousand-acre garden is home to several thousand species of plants, and their scientists are actively working with approximately four hundred medicinal species. Experts at the Central Siberian Botanical Garden have published over four thousand scientific papers and have contributed directly to new drug discovery and development from plants. The garden is home to botanists, phytochemists, and experts in all aspects of plant science. Since it is the central repository of botanical knowledge in all of Siberia, the botanical garden made an ideal first stop.

Sitting in the expansive office of the main building, I asked Director Vyacheslav Sedelnikov about the scope of medicinal plants in central Siberia. "We have hundreds of plants used as medicines in this region," he explained. "We have investigated many of these plants for their specific healing compounds, and we also know a great deal about how they grow, and the very best methods to maximize their potency. We have worked on drug development, and we have a lot of information that we are willing to share." I asked about *Rhodiola rosea.* "Ah yes, well, Rhodiola is one of the most beneficial plants in Siberia and very widely used. It is especially good for fighting stress, and it helps people to recover from fatigue and weakness due to illness. Plus we know that the root and its preparations are valuable aids to athletes. We have *Rhodiola rosea* right here in our gardens, which I will show you." When I asked Vyacheslav about the sexual properties of *Rhodiola rosea,* he broke into a smile at my question. "Here in Siberia, everybody knows about Rhodiola as an aphrodisiac. If a person has lost their desire or their ability to make love, *Rhodiola rosea* can restore them to healthy function. It is our very best plant for sexual vigor. It is truly one of the most effective of all plants."

Vera Cheryomushkina, Chief of the Laboratory for Medicinal and Aromatic plants, and Galina Vysochina, Chief of Phytochemistry, concurred with the director. "*Rhodiola rosea* is one of the most beneficial of all plants," Galina declared to me. "Because it is so popular, we have studied it a great deal." In fact, the two pointed out, *Rhodiola rosea* is Siberia's most highly treasured medicinal plant, and has been the subject of more scientific study and scrutiny than any other plant in that entire vast region. The plant is the subject of more than 180 phytochemical, pharmacological, and clinical published studies, most of them of Russian origin. Many of these studies were reported 2002 in issue 56 of *HerbalGram,* the journal of the American Botanical Council. That issue featured the most comprehensive overview of *Rhodiola rosea* ever published in English, enabling researchers in the United States to gain a well-informed understanding of this Siberian plant.

The trio produced a large volume containing at least a couple hundred maps of Siberia, showing the exact areas where *Rhodiola rosea* grows wild in abundance, with figures showing the tonnage that can be sustainably harvested from each region without damaging indigenous supply and habitat. The three areas in which the herb can be found in greatest abundance are the Altay, farther east in the Sayan Mountains, and in the region around Lake Baikal. As we studied the map, Vera pointed to those areas and commented "We have gone very far into this plant because of its significant value to health."

After cookies and tea and much conversation about plant medicines, we toured the various greenhouses at the Central Siberian Botanical Garden, housing their vast collections of flowering and tropical plants and their stunning collection of cacti. Outside, we toured several gardens of regional medicinal plants, arranged by health needs. Plants for headaches, respiratory health, cardiovascular health, and other purposes were grouped together. Director Sedelnikov smiled at my expressions of admiration. "You come back here with a TV crew and western scientists who are ready to collaborate with us. We have much to offer."

The Road to Altay

Marat and Vadim, their respective spouses, Rashida and Galina, and our driver Yevgeney and I headed off in a comfortable touring van to the Altay region, about 500 kilometers south of Novosibirsk. Our destination was remote Kuba, a small and scenic hamlet along the swift-running Katun River in a valley cut between steep, rocky mountains. There a rustic lodge would serve as our base of operations while we toured the Altay.

The trip took us through seemingly endless stretches of amber wheat, brilliant golden sunflowers, and vast patches of giant flowering *Cannabis sativa*, formerly used for hemp fiber and for the nutritional value of its seed. The plant is known more readily and commonly as marijuana. For hundreds of kilometers, everywhere I looked, whether in fields or private gardens, I saw great stands of tall cannabis. I requested that Yevgeney stop our bus innumerable times, so I could go running off into some fragrant cannabis thicket, to take close-up photographs of the tall, bushy specimens before me. In fact, they were of poor smoking quality, but they could supply an immense amount of fiber and seeds to the burgeoning hemp product market.

As we entered the Altay, I was struck by the majestic beauty of the place, which resembled the Austrian Alps and northern Vermont. Great rivers rushed swift and wide, huge hawks wheeled in the sky, and the air smelled fresh and sweet. Siberia was not what I had previously imagined. The views before me dispelled any Eisenhower-era notions that this was a dismal place. Leather-skinned horsemen tended herds of cattle and sheep, and grand mountain slopes with forests of pine and birch rose up around us as we wound our way through pristine valleys.

Along the road, we saw small stands where Altay people sold various herbal teas and preparations. We stopped at several stands and bought tea, honey, and herbs. One of the most popular of all preparations was *Rhodiola rosea* root, cut and and placed in a bottle, infused with vodka to extract and preserve it. I asked a woodsman about the Rhodiola drink. "Everybody I know uses Rhodiola regularly," he told me. "It keeps us alive. The root makes you very strong." I sampled a small mouthful of the drink and felt an immediate bracing effect. I bought a bottle for the trip. The woodsman smiled at me. "One time I was stranded in the woods in a bad storm for three days. I had only Rhodiola root in my pocket. The Rhodiola, plus some snow, kept me alive."

Siberia's Great Healer

No trip along the medicine trail would be complete without at least one visit to a distinguished traditional healer: the traditional herbalists and folk doctors know the uses of indigenous plant medicines best. We headed to the town of Gorno Altaisk, to meet with Siberia's most beloved herbal healer of all, Uri Vladimirovich. His modest apartment was crammed from one end to the other with fragrant herbs and preparations. Two younger female assistants helped him to package the herbs that, at seventy-seven, he still collects by hand, hiking the hills and mountains of the Altay. Uri possessed the kind eyes of a man who has spent his life engaged in good works that benefit others. Known throughout Russia, Uri is a celebrated keeper of the herbal flame. He welcomed us generously and appeared pleased by our company.

"My grandmother lived deep in the *taiga*, the forest," Uri explained. "She knew all the plants in her area, and she understood how to use them for healing. So when I was a young boy, I learned a lot from her. She would take me into the woods to gather plants. And she would also show me how to prepare them, and which plants to combine for different purposes. So that was the beginning of my herbal knowledge. My grandmother was the best teacher I could ever have. Then later as a young soldier in World War II, I was stationed in Greece, Macedonia, Bulgaria, and along the Black Sea. Those were very hard years. But in every region I sought out local herbal healers, and I learned about the plants. I spent time in the countryside whenever I could, and I found many valuable plants. So in this way, over time, I learned a great deal. After the war I became a geologist and traveled far and wide for my work. Everywhere

I went, I learned about plants and collected them. This went on for many years. After a while, I knew so much about herbs and was helping so many people, I no longer had time for geology. I left that behind and devoted myself entirely to healing with the plants given by nature."

The author of several books, including *Miracle Herbs of the Altay* and *Major Herbs of the Altay,* Uri was definitive when I inquired about *Rhodiola rosea.* "That herb is one of the very most important. It gives great strength, and it will help you to regain energy. Rhodiola also helps to fight stress. In this way it builds very good health. If you are sick, *Rhodiola* will help you to recover."

But what about the sexual effects of *Rhodiola,* I asked Uri.

"Ah, you bring up one of its most common uses. It is surely the greatest agent for sexual vigor. I have seen many people who suffer sexual trouble because of sickness or some other cause. They take *Rhodiola rosea,* and within a short while they regain their desire and their ability to have sex. I think that it is the very best thing for sex."

I asked if Uri had personally treated cases of lost libido and impotence with Rhodiola.

"Oh, yes, so many times. *Rhodiola* is extremely effective." He added that the root is also widely used by those who are sexually healthy as well. "It is traditional for couples to receive a bouquet of *Rhodiola rosea* roots on their wedding night, as a gift of love. This is common here in the Altay. They use the root, and they want to make love many times. Plus, *Rhodiola rosea* increases fertility. We have known this for a long time."

Uri showed us many of the herbal formulas he prepared for the people who seek his counsel. "They come here from all over Russia," he noted. "Even many people come from other countries. I have had visitors from many parts of Europe. They are sick, and they hear about me, they come and I help them. Some want to learn from me. So naturally I share whatever I can. Nature provides whatever we need to be healthy and alive. There is always a plant which can improve a person's condition."

I was deeply honored to meet such a kind and gentle healer as Uri Vladimirovich. He exemplifies the dedication and astute knowledge of the greatest specialists in natural plant medicines.

King of the Altay

Our travels around Gorno Altaisk led us to Haren Baludyan, a larger-than-life, boisterous herbal trader and founder of Narena Herbal Company, which distributes Siberian herbal tea formulas throughout Russia and to parts of Europe. Full of clever ideas almost to the point of bursting, Haren proudly declared early on, "I am King of the Altay." It may have been tempting to dismiss the claim as bluster, but in the few days we spent in Haren's company, he did seem to know everybody we encountered, and they all treated him with respect, warmth, and deference. The Altay did seem to be Haren's playground and kingdom. At one point I mentioned to Haren that he seemed to know everybody. Flashing a toothy grin, he countered, "No, they all know me."

A former teacher of mathematics and physics, Haren realized at one point that "I was never going to feed my family with mathematics!" He abruptly terminated his career in academia and turned his boundless energy to the emerging herb business, becoming an extraordinarily well-connected herbal trader in the Altay. He also started the largest bakery in Gorno Altaisk, because, as he explained, "There are 60,000 people here, and they all eat bread."

Haren offered to be of any possible service to the cause of my research. "What do you want? What do you need to see? Who do you want to meet? You tell me, and I will arrange it all, just like that." I took him up on the offer, and he proved true to his word.

"For starters," I said, "I would like to go all around this region to see as many of the local medicinal plants as you can show me. I would like to travel with some local plant experts and to go high up into the hills and see *Rhodiola rosea*. I will need samples of many plants, and I would like a list of the various regional plants and what they are used for."

Haren shrugged and gave a dismissive wave. "That is all? I thought that perhaps you would at least give me a challenge. Oh, well, it is no matter. We will meet tomorrow morning. You will have all of what you have requested, and a few extras thrown in. Now let us go have coffee and cookies."

Surely enough, early the next day we met with Haren, his driver Ashot, a local herb hunter named Anatoley, a woman botanist named Ira, and a plant collector named Olga. Once we were all assembled and had made brief introductions, Haren took charge like a superior officer directing his troops. "We will go now," Haren announced, pulling me into his car. Speeding along the narrow Altay roads from one majestic location to another, our three-car caravan motored into remote valleys, where we stopped to venture out into fields and woods, and up into high passes. Along the way, my companions spoke excitedly about the various plants we were viewing and their uses. The Siberian Altay is a center of incalculable botanical riches.

At one point Anatoley took me to a patch of plants with slender leaf-covered stalks and now dead flowers. *"Rhodiola rosea,"* he explained. He dug a plant up and invited me to smell the root. The root smelled like a fresh bouquet of highly fragrant roses. Thus the species name *rosea*. Anatoley pointed to the mountains around us. "Much more up there. That is the place to collect, up high."

Our group spent a delightful day moving from one zone to another, finally stopping by a river where we built a huge fire and enjoyed a barbeque. We sat in the warm afternoon sun and talked about the local herbs, and how everyone in the Altay uses and collects them. I asked the group more about *Rhodiola rosea*. Ira the botanist told me that it was the most widely collected of all plants in the region. "It is very popular, because it gives you great strength and energy," explained Anatoley the herb hunter. "Every woodsman and hunter and fisherman uses Rhodiola. It will help you to endure harsh conditions. It has a lot of life. I know people who have survived being trapped in blizzards by eating the root." The others confirmed that *Rhodiola rosea* lives up to its reputation. They all personally collected and used the plant.

I asked the group about the sexual effects of *Rhodiola rosea*. Haren laughed loudly and made a tight fist. "It makes your penis like hard wood!" Olga felt obliged to tell me that the majority of Altay village people use *Rhodiola rosea* as a matter of course, and that anybody who is middle-aged takes preparations of the root to stay in youthful sexual condition. The other men spoke of the sex-boosting properties of *Rhodiola rosea*. "You take plenty of Rhodiola, and I will find you a very nice woman," Haren proclaimed loudly. In my experience, any herb that enjoys such a long and widespread history of use as a sexual stimulant invariably proves effective. Often the question of how it works takes years or decades of chemical and clinical unraveling. Yet the plant demonstrates sexual potency-enhancing properties nonetheless. Hot plants come with the endorsement of millions of satisfied users.

At one point Haren pushed me in the ribs, a big grin on his face. "What did I tell you? I said I can arrange everything. Now you see for yourself. You want experts and herbs, and knowledge, and to see it for yourself, and it is as easy as a snap of the fingers." He wagged an index finger in midair. Are you satisfied now?" I laughed out loud and gave him a push back on the shoulder, and told him yes, and that just maybe he was in fact the King of the Altay. We all sat around the fire and ate and drank and told stories, until the Siberian sun began to slide close to the horizon.

Journey to the Source

My requests weren't finished. I wanted to go high up into the mountains, to hike to the prime spots where herb hunters collected *Rhodiola rosea*. On an overcast and chilly morning, Marat, Vadim, and I set off high up in windblown Semensky Pass in the company of an herb hunter named Yevgeney, yet another contact made by Haren. At around 2,500 meters, Semensky Pass isn't breathtakingly high, but a frigid wind and sleet made our hiking cold and wet. As we looked out at the gloom and frigid fog of the hike ahead, Marat asked, "Are you sure we need to go?" I told him yes, I had come a long way, and that rain or shine, I wanted to see the best growing areas of *Rhodiola rosea,* and to take pictures. I had two cameras, and

several rolls of film, and was ready to shoot. We set off res-
olutely into the gusty cold, as small hail blew into the necks of
our jackets.

Only a few kilometers along the trail, we encountered a
group of wild horses. The horses had sleek coats and powerful,
well-defined muscles. They stood eating a patch of plants I
thought I recognized. "That's *Rhaponticum*," noted Yevgeney
with a laugh. Second only to *Rhodiola rosea* in popularity,
Rhaponticum carthamoides is used by locals for stamina, and
by athletes for its ability to increase lean muscle mass. Yevgeney pointed to the horses. "They like Rhaponticum very
much. In the harvest season, we try to get to the plants before
the horses do. But they beat us to many of the plants." As we
hiked along higher and farther out, we warmed up and hit our
stride. "All over here we collect *Rhaponticum* and *Rhodiola*,"
Yevgeney told us. "But I will take you over a couple of valleys,
where the most plants can be found."

At the top of the pass, we made our way through tundra,
with its characteristic wet peat and low brush. Hidden rocks
slowed our progress, and the sky intermittently spat rain and
sleet. Still, the views were magnificent, with long expanses of
mountains and valleys, one after another, stretching to the
horizon. Eventually we came down into a valley, where Yevgeney pointed out hundreds of *Rhodiola rosea* plants. Marat
and Vadim smiled with relief. I was very pleased that I had insisted on traveling to the source to see for myself. There we
were, up in the mountains of Siberia, surrounded by one of the
most valuable plants in all of Asian traditional medicine.

Yevgeney showed us how to dig the roots of *Rhodiola rosea*.
Using a sharp piece of iron, he pulled up a couple of specimens.

I took plenty of photographs as I always do. When it finally got too cold to linger, we headed back, down the long path to where we had left our car. Once there, we turned on the heater, shed wet boots, and took big slugs of vodka infused with Rhodiola. "It's very important to use the plants," I announced in a professorial tone. We all laughed, from the joke, the vodka, and the relief of being warm again.

How Science Weighs In

I spent about two weeks in the company of Marat and Vadim, their wives Rashida and Galina, our driver Yevgeney, and a host of plant experts from all around the Altay. Once back in the States, I delved into the extensive body of science that exists on *Rhodiola rosea*. We overuse words like remarkable and miraculous, until they are just mere superlatives in a language awash with hyperbole. In fact, *Rhodiola rosea* proves to be one of the most broadly beneficial, superbly healing, restorative, and sexually enlivening plants on earth. It is nothing short of miraculous.

Rhodiola rosea contains a group of novel compounds that have not been found in other plants. These include rosin, rosavin, and rosarin, known collectively as "rosavins." Each of these has been studied, and each appears to make a significant contribution to the plant's unrivaled antistress properties. Rhodiola also contains the agent salidroside and protective antioxidants that inhibit the cellular deterioration process of oxidation, which is akin to rusting.

One of the great advances in more widespread understanding of *Rhodiola rosea* occurred when the journal of the American Botanical Council, *HerbalGram,* published an overview on *Rhodiola rosea* in 2002. This outstanding piece of work drew from more than one hundred previously untranslated Russian studies on the plant and its effects on health, revealing it to be a potent and versatile natural healer. Coauthored by preeminent *Rhodiola* scholar Zakir Ramazanov and New York psychiatrists Richard Brown and Patricia Gerbarg, their report detailed *Rhodiola rosea*'s proven benefits for the nervous, endocrine, cardiovascular, and reproductive systems, as well as anticancer effects. The overview also described cases of improved mental and emotional health due to *Rhodiola rosea* use, in patients who had not benefited from other interventions, including drugs and pscyhotherapy.

Rhodiola rosea is one of a handful of plants that fits the criteria of adaptogens, those agents that promote nonspecific resistance to a wide range of adverse influences of all kinds, including harmful factors that are physical, biological, and chemical. As an adaptogen, *Rhodiola rosea* helps to reestablish normal, healthy function under conditions of stress ranging from mild to severe. This is exactly where the plant's sexual effects kick in.

Under stress, many different compounds increase in the body, including adrenaline, opioids, and catecholamine. If levels of these substances remain high in the system, they can produce damage to nervous and glandular function, including the sex glands. One substance, CRF, or corticotrophin releasing factor, has been studied extensively. CRF increases in the body as a result of stress and can in time lead to impaired sexual function. CRF actually promotes an additional feeling of stress, perpetuating an already taxing condition. Commonly, this is accompanied by a feeling of overall fatigue, characterized by mental fatigue in particular. In studies, *Rhodiola rosea* has been shown to reduce various stress-induced chemicals in the body to normal levels, and alleviate general and mental fatigue. *Rhodiola* lowers levels of CRF specifically, enabling the body and mind to recuperate and establish normal function. In cases of stress-induced loss of libido and diminished sexual function, *Rhodiola rosea* can help to bring the near dead back to vibrant life.

While *Rhodiola rosea* is the subject of a number of successful Russian human clinical studies, two sexual studies stand out. Among forty women who suffered amenorrhea (loss of menses), daily administration of *Rhodiola rosea* extract for two weeks restored menses. Subsequently, eleven of the women became pregnant. Among thirty-five men with erectile dysfunction, twenty-six experienced significantly improved sexual function, as a result of taking *Rhodiola rosea* extract for three months. Additionally, the men experienced normalization of prostatic fluid. Rhodiola rosea restores healthy sexual function in many cases.

More important for our purposes, beyond a few dozen people involved in human clinical studies, a multitude of Siberian people have used *Rhodiola rosea* for centuries. The root is hailed as an exceptional sex enhancer. In the Altay region, every man and woman I met used *Rhodiola rosea* regularly. All were clear about its sex-enhancing virtues. Stress ages us, robbing us of our youth and our youthful sexuality. *Rhodiola rosea* combats the systemic effects of stress, reversing some dimensions of the aging process, reinvigorating our sexual functions.

Using *Rhodiola rosea*

You can experience *Rhodiola rosea* in a few ways. You can travel to the Siberian Altay and swig *Rhodiola rosea* from a woodsman's vodka bottle, or you can use the root in fluid or powdered extract supplement forms. I enjoy fluid extracts of the root, because I like its rosy aroma and astringent flavor. In human clinical studies, a standardized powdered extract was used in many cases. That extract was standardized to 3 percent rosavins and 0.8 percent salidroside. This is information you look for on a product label.

Participants in studies took between 150–200 milligrams of the extract daily. You can find such standardized extract supplements in natural product stores. Look in the resource section at the back of this book for preferred brands.

Stress is a killer, there's no doubt about it. And the sexual toll that stress can exact is awful. But nature offers a hot plant that restores vigor, banishes fatigue, improves strength, and helps to reinvigorate sexual appetite and function. That plant, *Rhodiola rosea,* is a titan of natural sexual healing power.

HEART OF DARKNESS

Pausinystalia yohimbe

ON A HOT, STICKY MAY NIGHT IN ACCRA, GHANA, I SAT UNDER a starry sky, enraptured by a group of African musicians and dancers. The dozen performers gave a show that was at once dynamic, polyrhythmic, and infectiously exciting in its hip-shaking, butt-wiggling, breast-jiggling celebration of life. Four drummers beat out ingenious rhythms that mingled and flowed fast and slow, alternating between the slow heartbeat of the jungle and the rapid, pulsating beat of Carnival.

The three striking women dancers in the group stood short, medium and tall, each one taking turns as the featured performer, accentuating the moves of her performance with her bodily shape. The tallest of the three possessed a Grace Jones angularity and moved in a sultry, leopardlike manner, relying on the smooth flow of her long legs and arms to convey an essential sexuality. The more full-figured medium-height dancer thrust and bounced the mounds of her bottom in a manner utterly astonishing for her pneumatic speed and precision control. The shortest of the dancers moved with erotic and suggestive undulations similar to the second, but my attention was

immediately drawn to her feet. Barefoot like the other performers, she slapped her feet flat on the ground with well-articulated
precision, yet soundlessly, as though right at the point of im-
pact, an insulating air cushion silenced the percussion of her
soles on the patio tile on which she moved.

The vibrant group performed traditional songs and dances
from Ghana, Ivory Coast, Senegal, and Burkina Faso, pounding
out tribal rhythms and singing and dancing late into the night.
Throughout the evening, they exclaimed spontaneously with
great vigor as they carried on. It was my first night in Ghana,
and the steamy sensuality of the performance seemed a marvelous way to begin my exploration of a highly prized African
hot plant, yohimbe.

I had traveled to Ghana, a West African country with rapidly
diminishing rainforest, to investigate several plants, especially
yohimbe. Of all the world's hot plants, yohimbe is among the
very best known. Found in the forests of Nigeria, Cameroon,
Gabon, Congo, and Ghana, yohimbe (*Pausinystalia yohimbe*) is a
tall evergreen that reaches a height of twenty-five meters. The
bark of the tree contains a group of alkaloids, most notably
yohimbine, which makes up as much as 6 percent of the bark
by weight. Yohimbe, with a long history of folk use as an
aphrodisiac, is typically prepared by boiling shavings of the
bark and drinking the resulting decoction.

Yohimbine, the primary alkaloid found in yohimbe bark is a
known fast-acting central nervous system stimulant, with specific action upon the nerves of the lower spine. Yohimbine
causes dilation of the peripheral vessels of the corpus cavernosum, the erectile tissue that forms the dorsal and sides of the
penis. In plain words, the bark extract promotes a good, firm

erection. This penis-vessel-dilating activity has given yohimbine a well-deserved reputation as a sexual stimulant. An erection is the result of engorgement of the fine vessels of the corpus cavernosum, and yohimbe makes that engorgement occur. Voilà, an erection is born.

In women, yohimbine promotes increased circulation to the clitoris, promoting what some refer to as a "clitoral buzz." The stimulation produced by yohimbe in this manner makes the plant a very significant sexual stimulant for women as well as men, though typically men use yohimbe far more than women.

As far back as the 1890s, European physicians employed yohimbe to treat impotence. Today yohimbine hydrochloride is the active constituent in a number of over-the-counter and prescription sex drugs, including the brands Afrodex®, Aphrodyne®, Pluriviron®, Prowess®, Yocon®, Yohimex®, and Yohydrol®. The majority of yohimbe sells through the booming herbal supplement market, where users employ preparations of the bark for a sexual boost. Relatively inexpensive and fast-acting, yohimbe has earned a secure place in the market and a solid reputation as a hot plant. My task was to find out more about yohimbe in its natural and cultural home.

In the Market

The morning after the dance and music performance, I strolled along the streets of downtown Accra toward the Makola Market, my senses bombarded by a multitude of sights, sounds, and smells. At the edge of the sprawling market, I stood amid vendors selling leather goods, carved masks, wooden stools, fresh rustic bread, beaded necklaces, brightly colored fabrics, and local crafts. I had been there for only a minute when I was approached by a tall, striking-looking man with a shaved head and bare feet, and three tribal scars on each cheek. He introduced himself as Joseph, and offered to show me around. I liked his manner and agreed.

We passed unclad children playing, adults sleeping under trees, and mothers squatting in the dirt. The full experience of Ghana's poverty could be witnessed readily on the street, where thousands struggled to earn a meager wage to buy a small bit of food each day. Women carried high stacks of bread on their heads, and others performed remarkable cranial balancing acts with bags of sugar, flour, cloth, large buckets of smoked fish, and other goods. Several cab drivers honked and made gestures indicating that their cabs were empty, but I waved them off, content to walk the dusty packed street with Joseph, sweating beneath the hot equatorial sun.

As we moved deeper into the market, we negotiated our way around open sewers, on both sides of which vendors sold flip-flops, buckets of nails, dried whole fish, raw meat, pudding, sugar, peanuts, inner tubes, bicycle chains, pork skins, hot peppers, ground spices, breads, T-shirts, cloth, flour, vegetables, pots and pans, and decorative shells. High-life music blared from oversize boom boxes and from absurdly large speakers set upon crates. The strong smell of cooking food mixed with the cloying aroma of garbage and sewage, all of it baking under the unrelenting midday sun. Muddy trickles of stinking, milky-looking water ran into fetid depressions, while battered old cars banged through the deep ruts of the market roads, kicking up swirling clouds of fine, light brown dust, which settled like talc upon everything. Large vultures wheeled overhead in slow, lazy circles, waiting for anything, or anyone, to die.

I explained to Joseph that I wished to see any medicinal plants being sold, in any form. "You want to see the traditional medicines, I know exactly where to take you," Joseph told me with confidence. We made our way around sleeping dogs, dodged naked running children between stalls, and passed men playing checkers on vegetable crates. After a time, we came to a row of tables where men and women displayed a wide variety of dried barks, berries, roots, and leaves, as well as herbal preparations in bottles and jars and bins. As it turned out, Joseph knew more than a little about the regional herbal medicines of the area. He spoke with a number of the vendors and explained to me what I was looking at and what various herbs were for. He picked up a small handful of bark and asked, "You know yohimbe?" I told him that I was especially interested in yohimbe. He related that to the vendor who displayed the bark, and that led to some good-natured banter about the sexual power of yohimbe.

At the next table, another man announced to us that he also had yohimbe for sale. We moved along and spoke with him awhile. "I have seen many men use this bark with very good results," said the man in good English. I asked how the bark was usually prepared, and the vendor, whose name was Edgar, said that boiling the bark for an hour or so and consuming the resulting tea was the best way to derive its benefits. Edgar made the universal sign of a sturdy erection with his arm and made a comment about yohimbe helping a man to have sex with many women. Then Joseph announced proudly that he didn't need any yohimbe, or anything else for that matter, to have sex with many women. I inquired whether there was any more popular sex plant in that region. No, Edgar and Joseph told me, yohimbe was king. But there wasn't as much as there used to be, Edgar said with sadness. "A lot of the trees are gone, and much of the forest is gone, too."

At one time, all of West Africa was covered with equatorial rain forest, but only small remnants of the forests remain, as clearing for grazing, timber, and human sprawl have whittled the forests down to a fraction of their former size. Incalculable numbers of plant, animal, and insect species have been lost forever. The land, once moist forest floor hosting a riot of lush green vegetation, became hard brown dust, barely nutritious enough to support the most sparse crop life. The deforestation of Africa, as elsewhere, is a sad tale of environmental devastation caused by a series of ill-considered actions.

After speaking with various herbal vendors in Makola Market, Joseph and I headed to a small, shaded outdoor bar, where we drank some cold Star Beer, brewed in Accra. The dewy bottle felt refreshing against my sweaty, dusty face. Joseph spoke about himself. He was trained as a computer programmer in Lagos, Nigeria, where he grew up. "I like to associate with business people, smart people, you know. There was no work for me in Lagos, so I came here, and now I sell some traditional crafts. Also, I take people around. This is business for me, and I also meet good people." Joseph went on to explain that he knew all the best places in and around Accra, and that he could be of help to me.

The most intriguing part of our conversation came when Joseph informed me that his father, now deceased, had been a highly talented herbalist. Throughout his childhood, Joseph learned about medicinal plants and their uses through his father.

"He was very intelligent," Joseph told me with pride. "My father knew the plants very well, and he taught me about them." That explained Joseph's apparent familiarity with the plant medicines in the market. Joseph told me about a number of plants with especially significant healing properties as we drank cold beer in the sweltering hot shade.

Where the Elephants Hide

About thirty kilometers north of Cape Coast, the Kakum Rainforest Preserve sits like an emerald jewel amid Ghana's ocean of dry brown dust. The last of the country's once vast rain forest, the three-hundred-fifty-square-kilometer Kakum afforded an excellent opportunity to see West African plant life in its natural primeval habitat. The ride would take a couple of hours from Accra, and so I found a friendly looking driver named Fred, who was happy to take me to Kakum, happy for the work.

Riding out of the crowded and chaotic city, we traveled along a coastal road packed with trucks, cars, a few buses, and occasional motorcycles. Goats, chickens, children, and adults also occupied the narrow two lanes, greatly slowing our driving progress while improving the sightseeing. The farther we traveled outside of Accra, the more rustic the landscape became as we passed through the small towns of Bortianor, Kokokrobite, Nyanyaano, Awut, and Winneba. In those places, most buildings were constructed of mud with palm thatch roofs.

Between villages people readied the land for planting crops, employing the soil-destroying slash-and-burn method. The villagers cut away vegetation with a hand machete, and then set the brush and grass on fire. We passed one angry blaze after another, high red flames leaping in the air and licking at the vegetation, leaving smouldering charred ground. The air was thick with smoke, and we spotted some very large hillside blazes from miles away. Fred commented on the hellish scene. "The people are preparing the land. They burn it, then the rains come and they will plant." The people do not comprehend that the destructive method of small-crop farming has created the endless sea of dust in which they live.

The coastal road bustled with commerce. Women sold corn, pudding, salt, bread, and fish. Neat piles of water coconuts stood on display at tiny wooden stands, ready to quench the thirst of hot travelers. Some women sat with large stacks of fresh pineapples. Fred saw those and remarked, "Oh, they are so sweet, so sweet, and juicy." We stopped and I bought a couple of pineapples, which were every bit as good as Fred had claimed.

We passed stands of sugarcane and village markets set up with slat wood fences and tables. When we passed a man holding up a dead animal by the tail, I asked Fred what it was. "A grass cutter," he replied. Does it taste good? "Oh, yes, very good, tender." Shortly after, a man stood at the side of the road holding up another animal. "Antelope," Fred remarked. "People have nothing to do, no jobs, so they go into the forest and hunt animals and then sell them for money." We passed several men holding up animals in the approximate shape of large tennis rackets, which turned out to be grass cutters which had been gutted, stretched on sticks and smoked. They looked very much like roadkill armadillo after too many truck tires and too much hot sun.

After a couple of hours we approached the lush green forest of Kakum, which is home to several hundred species of birds, over six thousand species of insects, four hundred types of but-terflies, monkeys, bongo, antelope, river hogs, and numerous varieties of snakes, including vipers like the king cobra and the green mamba. Most notably, Kakum is also home to the elu-sive forest elephants. At a lodge I met with a short slim guide named Rockson, who wore an outfit with a Ghana Forestry Ser-vice patch on his shirt. I explained that I wanted to hike deep into Kakum, and that I wished to see medicinal plants, notably yohimbe. Rockson smiled at the mention of the sex tree. "Yes, we can go for a long way. The forest is filled with many plants that we use for medicines, and I can show them to you. But we cannot remove any samples, because this is a preserve, and we protect all species here." Rockson's English was impeccable and I readily agreed to the conditions he described.

Rockson and I walked from the forest lodge about one kilo-meter up a road, where we reached a trail head. "From here we go into the forest." He commented, "Stay with me. We must be careful." As we made our way through the thick, humid growth of the forest, I was happy to be wearing sturdy boots, rip-resistant pants, and a shirt. Thorny lianas snagged us, ground vines tripped our feet, and muddy inclines made for slow walk-ing. The forest was rich with concentrated oxygen and heavy with a thousand aromas. Some smells were musty, some fecal, some sweet, some fresh and green. Insects buzzed, fluttered, hummed, and whizzed. Birds chirped, cawed, trilled, and squawked. Monkeys leapt and called from the canopy high above, and parrots made a racket. We entered one small area where the air was thick with hundreds of tiny fluttering laven-der butterflies.

Not that far into the forest Rockson pointed out the first yohimbe tree. It stood about eighty feet tall and was quite broad at the top. "Here these trees are protected," Rockson commented. "But in other places, people cut them down, because they are worth money." I admired the yohimbe tree, and asked Rockson if he knew a lot about yohimbe. "Most people know about it. If you want to have sex when you are older, or if you have some kind of sexual trouble, then often yohimbe will help. It is very popular among men."

During our hike in the forest, we saw several tall yohimbe trees. I was glad to see them in their natural habitat and to take some photographs. At one point, Rockson stopped on the path as a green mamba, one of the poisonous snakes in the forest, slithered by just feet away from us. "Good thing it is not black instead," Rockson said. He was referring to Africa's deadly and highly aggressive black mamba, which strikes to kill with blinding speed. We heard many monkeys overhead, but saw only the fleeting shapes of a few, as they screeched and leapt from one tree to another, high up in the canopy. Suddenly, the forest around us became very quiet, and we caught a flash of something very large and brown ahead of us, melting soundlessly into the forest, swallowed by the greenery. "Forest elephant," Rockson pointed. Though I had heard that the forest elephants of West Africa were quiet, I assumed that I would hear them because of their size. But the elephant that disappeared in front of us moved as soundlessly as an owl. "We are very lucky," Rockson told me. "It is hard to see the elephants at all." The forest elephant is erroneously referred to as the "Pygmy elephant" because it is smaller than the savannah elephant. The two are in fact separate species. I was happy to know that even as the rain forest was diminishing, large wild creatures still roamed there.

After a day of mostly pathless threading through the forest,

Rockson led us to the Kakum canopy walkway, which is unique in all of Africa. The suspended canopy walkway is composed of over 300 meters of swinging bridge and six tree-trunk-mounted platforms, which reach heights of 100 meters. The walkway was designed to depend entirely upon trees for support, with no nails or bolts used. Instead, steel cables were carefully wrapped around trunks to provide the necessary stabilization. Above the trees of Kakum, I was able to view the vast expanse of the forest preserve. The vista was stunning. Birds by the hundreds flew between the trees and I spotted monkeys leaping about.

The Doctor's Opinion

On a blazing hot morning I met at my hotel with Dr. Quaynor of Agrata Herbs and his right-hand man, Samuel Ofou. A naturopathic physician, Quaynor operated three clinics, in Accra, Cape Coast, and Takoradi. He claimed a total of 12,000 patients, which I assumed represented the total number of patient visits in his career. "I have a vision to provide natural health care to many, many people. I can offer fine herbal remedies which will assist people to restore harmony within themselves." Quaynor was a man on a mission, and he wanted me to visit his herbal manufacturing business straight away. We departed the hotel, piled into a small blue pickup truck, and headed off across town along rutted, poorly kept roads.

When we arrived at Quaynor's Agrata Herbs in a small, quiet neighborhood, his four-year-old daughter ran up to him and threw her arms tightly around his knees with wild enthusiasm. Then she did the same to me. I patted her head, and she ran off happy and laughing. Quaynor and Samuel took me to a modest building where they hand-filled six thousand bottles of herbal extracts of various types every week. Large glass vessels contained herbs undergoing extraction in a solution of alcohol and water. Stacks of boxes filled with bottles were lined up against the walls. I was impressed by their level of production in the cramped, rather rudimentary facility. Samuel explained, "We have so many people who want herbal remedies. Even though we are quite small, we make a lot of products, and this helps so many people with their health."

I asked Quaynor and Samuel about yohimbe. "It is very useful," Quaynor remarked. "We are extracting some right now in this container." He pointed to a large vessel in which a large pile of tree bark was soaking. "Yohimbe is especially good for men, for sexual performance. Sometimes a man cannot achieve an erection. If this is the case, then often yohimbe can help." Samuel showed me the labels of an herbal product in which yohimbe was a main ingredient. "For men," he told me, holding his right hand in a tight fist. "It makes men hard."

Quaynor and Samuel explained that they hoped to expand their operation, and that they had drawn up a business plan to supply to any potential investors. They both described to me how difficult it was to conduct business in Ghana, and they expressed their sincere belief that Ghana's herbal wealth could open up rich opportunity for many people in that country, with some development dollars and a better understanding of good business practices. I see this all over the world. Many native people know the true value of their traditional plant remedies and are often thwarted in their efforts to grow businesses, due to lack of funds and an inadequate understanding of commerce. Trade in traditional plant medicines can infuse a poor economy with a steady stream of trade dollars and can provide jobs for many people who very much want to work.

Voucher Samples

That afternoon a friendly driver named Henry picked me up at my hotel in a faded and somewhat dented Audi. I liked Henry so much he remained my driver for another week. Negotiating slow traffic on wretchedly damaged roads, Henry set a course for the University of Accra, which occupied a large campus outside of the city. At the university I set off to find Daniel Abbiw, director of the Ghana Herbarium, where specimens of plants are held as reference samples, also known as voucher specimens. These specimens are used to corroborate the identity of plants when needed. Voucher samples are pressed and arranged in files, in a librarylike system.

Several people offered completely contradictory locations for the herbarium. But after more than an hour of intensive hunting around on a sprawling campus, I gathered sufficient information to find it. In a dim hall I located botanical expert Daniel Abbiw, author of *Useful Plants of Ghana*. Abbiw proved to have a wealth of knowledge about Ghanaian plants, and about the country's traditional people and their customs. Abbiw not only directed the herbarium and wrote books on medicinal plants, but he also worked with Vicdoris Pharmaceuticals, probably the largest exporter of Ghanaian and other African herbs. "I help the companies to know exactly how much there is of a certain plant, and I make sure that the identification is also correct."

I asked Daniel to show me a voucher sample of yohimbe. He

led me to a large metal filing cabinet and found the sample in short order. Various parts of the tree, proper botanical name, the date, and location where the sample was taken were all included in the file. I asked about yohimbe. "It is not so abundant now," he told me. "Any time you have a popular plant, it must be managed correctly. But yohimbe is very popular, and there is money to be made from harvesting the trees. So it is now in short supply in Ghana, because it has been overharvested. If someone would develop a plantation, they could produce a lot of material, and it would also prove highly profitable, I'm sure." Daniel Abbiw clearly understood the need for the development of a medical-plant agriculture industry in Ghana.

What the Human Studies Show

Though women have reportedly used yohimbe, men use it most frequently, for its functional enhancement of erections. To date there are no human clinical studies on whole yohimbe bark or bark extract, but there are ten human clinical studies on yohimbine, the active consituent in yohimbe bark. Now that standardized extracts of yohimbe bark can offer specific doses of yohimbine, you can use the bark extract, available as an herbal supplement, instead of the purified drug. And yohimbine hydrochloride is indeed a drug, one of many pharmaceutical agents derived from plants and sold by prescription.

Yohimbine has been tested against placebo in ten randomized trials with 659 men. In the studies 335 men received yohimbine and 324 received a placebo. The results of the studies are good. Yohimbine provided satisfactory erections in 30 percent of men as compared with 14 percent with placebo. The dose of yohimbine given in the studies ranged between 15 mg and 44 mg daily, for four to ten weeks of treatment. Erectile studies measure the ability to achieve an erection and firmness of erections. The time yohimbe takes to work depends on the man. Some experience quick results. With some, it takes days or weeks.

More studies will help to establish whether the specific cause of erectile dysfunction, age, or the severity of condition are related to the degree of benefit achieved with yohimbine. Keep in mind that studies have focused on erectile dysfunction. What about reasonably healthy, functional men who wish to add a little extra kick to their sex lives? This is, in fact, yohimbe's broadest use today. Standardized extracts of the bark are taken by healthy males for a sexual boost, with recommended doses ranging from 8 milligrams to 20 milligrams of yohimbine daily. More is not necessarily better with yohimbe. There is some clinical evidence showing that a lower dose of about 10 milligrams of yohimbine daily may do more to enhance sexual function than a higher dose.

Though yohimbe is generally safe for a majority of users, it causes rapid heartbeat, nervousness, sleeplessness, and hyperstimulation in some individuals. These unwanted side effects go away when the use of yohimbe is discontinued. Yohimbe should not be taken by people who have heart, liver, or kidney disease. Diabetics who wish to use yohimbe to improve erectile function should consult a physician before doing so. If you are taking an MAO-inhibiting drug, do not use yohimbe without first consulting your physician. Plants can interact with certain drugs, and yohimbe interacts with MAO inhibitors.

Jungle Fever

Word gets around a place like Ghana. A foreigner shows up, he's interested in plants, especially those which enhance sexual function, and there's a possibility of some commerce. Close to two dozen people showed up at my little hotel to tell me about their herbal products, or their connections to commercial quantities of plant materials. From antimalarials to novel sweeteners, people in Ghana have a lot to sell. I gathered an impressive pile of business cards and contact information to bring back to the United States.

One afternoon Joseph, the Nigerian I'd met early in my trip, showed up. We sat and had iced coffees in the shade, and he asked me if I would like to get together with him and some friends later that evening. "What's the occasion?" I asked. Joseph explained to me that he had told his friends about our walk through the Makola Market together and about my interest in plants. Some of his friends wanted to meet me, and they would like to arrange a meal and music and dancing. "Sure," I told him. "I'd love to go."

That evening Joseph reappeared. We got into Henry's Audi and headed north out of the city. It was just dusk, and the air was cooled down to very warm instead of roasting. Insects chirped loudly as we rode past large stands of tall grasses, leaving the city lights behind. I sat in the passenger seat, a warm wind blowing in my face. After about half an hour we came to a small neighborhood of houses. One had colorful lights strung from the roof to a tree, and I could hear upbeat music. Several people stood outside, some drinking beer. Two striking-looking women wore form-fitting outfits of kente cloth, a brilliantly colorful African cloth woven with dazzling designs. Both were tall, sleek, and tawny.

Joseph acted the perfect gentleman, making introductions all around. Two men were from Gabon, and most of the other men and women were Ghanaian. The two women were from Nigeria and apparently had known Joseph for a few years. Both were beautiful, and to my surprise and delight, they seemed interested in spending time with me. Estelle and Clara—to protect their privacy, pseudonyms have been used—were secretaries who worked in Accra. Speaking perfect English they were full of questions. How did I like Ghana? Was it my first time in Africa? Is it true that I was studying some sex plants? Did I think that women in Ghana were beautiful? Would I tell them what life is like in the United States? How long would I be staying? Was I married? I negotiated my way through the various questions, and they both took delight in my answers and laughed a lot and affectionately patted my shoulders. At various times, Estelle and Clara took my arms in theirs and led me to different places—to a cooler for a beer, to a garden to see some flowers, to the backyard to look up at emerging stars. It was a warm African night, and I was happily in the care of two charming women.

I made the rounds, chatting with everybody there. Joseph made sure that I had a chance to speak with everyone, though Estelle and Clara remained ever present, faithfully at my sides as though I were their charge. We ate chicken, local cooked vegetables, bread, and pineapple.

At one point, Joseph announced that he had something "special" for me. I was led to the kitchen, where Joseph handed me a small bottle of cloudy brown liquid. The contents looked like some sort of herbal decoction. Joseph pointed and smiled.

"Yohimbe. I got it for you in the market and made a strong tea so you can try it here." It seemed like a good idea. I tend to consume the herbs I study, according to the maxim that you can't know a plant until you use it. The herbal preparation was apparently ready for drinking. A man with whom I'd spoken earlier produced a cup. He then poured some of the liquid and gave it to me. "Strong," Joseph pointed out.

I began to sip. Like many bark teas, it tasted bitter, though not unpleasant. I moved around through the party with Estelle and Clara, slowly polishing off the cup of yohimbe tea. Within a few minutes I felt a lift and a sense of openness in my chest. I also felt just a bit flushed and quite energized. Someone turned the music up louder, and everybody began to dance. I enjoyed two dancing partners, Estelle and Clara. We danced until we were covered with sweat, until salty droplets of perspiration stung my eyes. At one point, Clara said "Come, you are hot. We will get you a cloth." The two women led me to a pretty and secluded patio.

Estelle and Clara did get the salt out of my eyes, and the sweat off my brow. Music played in the background, and insects chirping in the grass competed with the sounds of drums and guitars. I was more comfortable with my shirt off, and apparently so were they. It was good to be off my feet, and I could feel the yohimbe working through my system. We ate little pieces of chilled pineapple, and the two women laughed a lot. Moon shone down onto our private spot as we reclined. The night wore on, happily and delightfully.

Using Yohimbe

Look for Yohimbe products containing extracts standardized to specified levels of the alkaloid yohimbine. Consume between

8–20 milligrams of yohimbine daily, no more. In the instance of Yohimbe, a smaller amount of yohimbine (say 12 milligrams) may prove more effective than the larger 20 milligram dose. If you feel as though your heartbeat is becoming rapid, then better to reduce your dose. And if you feel tumescent and ready for love, then you are right where you want to be with this hot plant from the steaming rain forests of West Africa.

THE FEROCIOUS YIN YANG

Horny Goat Weed

ACCORDING TO ANCIENT LEGEND, THERE ONCE LIVED IN THE wilds of China's northern Szechuan province a remarkable beast known as the Yin Yang. This animal, it was said, was so ferociously sexual, it copulated one hundred times daily with great enthusiasm. The tremendous sexual vigor of the Yin Yang, and its olympian stamina, was reputedly due to the creature's diet. For the ferocious Yin Yang regularly ate the fresh green leaves of epimedium. Today, that once little-known plant from the mountains of China is increasingly popular in the United States by its folk name, horny goat weed. Far removed from the teapots of antiquity, this hot plant has burst upon the scene like a flash bomb. One horny goat weed formula has become one of the best-selling herbal supplements of all time. National magazine ads for the formula feature sultry women in skimpy attire lying across double-page spreads. Their eyes suggest mischief. The formula is boldly promoted for its lust-generating, performance-enhancing benefits. Horny goat weed—what an apt name!

How did this sizzling fever for a previously obscure herb

happen? Some of the important scientific references on plant medicine have for years mentioned various species of the herb epimedium for enhanced libido and improved sexual function. Botanist James Duke, one of the preeminent experts in the field of plant medicine, is most responsible for initiating the popularity of the aphrodisiac plant that sells like there's no tomorrow. In the 1990s, Dr. Duke, who enjoyed a long and distinguished career as the USDA's top plant expert, began speaking tó groups in the natural products industry. Dr. Duke shared his knowledge of medicinal plants at various gatherings, conferences, and conventions, attracting an enthusiastic and eclectic crowd very different from that of his governmental colleagues. Dr. Duke found attentive and enterprising admirers of his knowledge of traditional medicine, who listened closely for references to plants that might lead to new herbal products. When Jim Duke started to talk about epimedium by its folk name, horny goat weed, eyebrows raised. Duke said that horny goat weed was a true aphrodisiac. That was the tipping point.

It didn't take long before herbal companies in the United States tracked down and ordered Chinese species of horny goat weed. They found the herb well known among traders, moderately priced, and readily available. A horny goat weed groundswell began. No one could have predicted what would follow next. One of the people who took a keen interest in the herb was entrepreneur Mel Rich, whose New York company Phoenix Labs makes some of the most popular products on the market. A pharmacist by training, Mel knows how to dig into the background of an herb and verify its reputation and effects. He liked the sex claims for epimedium, and the herb passed his tests for legitimacy. He believed that the sex category was ready for a breakthrough herbal product that could attract more mainstream consumers than ever before. And he especially liked the folk name horny goat weed. It was perfect. He knew he could sell that. Mel developed an herbal fomula for sex enhancement called Horny Goat Weed, which combined epimedium from China, maca from Peru, *Mucuna pruriens* from India, and a species of Polypodium, and got it into national distribution through every GNC store. Within a short period of time, Horny Goat Weed was available in American malls from coast to coast. It was hard to miss the big, bold letters on the bottle. Horny Goat Weed started to sell.

Responding to Mel Rich's bold mass-market advertising and promotional campaign for Horny Goat Weed, millions of curious consumers into went to stores to try the formula. Mel had a runaway success on his hands. "Well you know," he remarked about the rising fortunes of Horny Goat Weed, "you try a lot of different things, and it takes so much effort just to get a product to market. Then you have no guarantee that it's going to sell well. So when something like this happens, in a way it's a vindication of other projects that maybe didn't necessarily do well for any number of reasons."

With Horny Goat Weed taking off like a rocket, Mel Rich realized that he needed to know even more about the plant and to better understand its place in the Chinese market. So he called me. As a medicine hunter, part of my job involves following the chain of trade, to understand any and all aspects of a plant, where it originates, and how it is traded. How much is there? Where is it sold? When is it harvested? By whom? My role is to garner the answers to these questions and more. The information I assemble helps a company to evaluate the market potential and circumstances of a plant, its supply, and availability.

As you have already learned, I meet with scientific, medical, and traditional experts in a plant's native country, most of whom are only too happy to share valuable information. There is a tremendous wealth of knowledge on plants. But it's in many different languages and the experts in the field are found all over. Mel needed as much field information as possible on horny goat weed. He asked me to organize a research trip in China to investigate. The herb was clearly on a fast market track.

Horny Goat Weed?

Known in Traditional Chinese Medicine (TCM) as Yin Yang Huo, the uses of epimedium or horny goat weed was first described in the two-thousand-year-old Chinese medicinal text *Shen Nong Ben Cao Jing*. Horny goat weed is any of several species of epimedium, including *Epimedium brevicorum, pubescens, sagittatum,* and *grandiflorum*. In TCM epimedium is used to restore sexual energy, treat impotence, increase production of semen, strengthen connective tissue such as bones, tendons, and muscles. Epimedium also is used for its antiarthritic activity, in cases of mental fatigue and poor memory, and to treat high blood pressure due to menopause.

A leafy perennial, epimedium grows profusely in the wild in the Chinese countryside, most abundantly at higher altitudes. The green leaves of the plant contain a variety of beneficial natural compounds, including flavonoids, polysaccharides, and icariin, which are presumed to be responsible for its effects.

Though the exact way that horny goat weed works remains unknown, studies show that the plant demonstrates activity similar to androgens, which are sex hormones that stimulate desire in men and women.

A Horny Goat Weed Expedition

To get inside the herbal scene in southern China, I needed the help of people who knew their way around. I made contact with several people in the herbal business, informing them of my upcoming trip. I planned to take notes on all aspects of horny goat weed harvesting and commerce, science and traditional use, and to shoot photographs as well. I sent a list of things I wanted to see and received confirmation that plans were being made for my arrival. One of my contacts was Jerry Wu, whose company Draco manufactures a number of Chinese herbal extracts, including horny goat weed. Jerry promised to help me achieve my objectives.

On every successful research trip, I need the help of willing individuals who will devote time, energy, and expertise to my pursuits. They stand to benefit through business, and so we share interests. The more I learn, the more I will communicate in articles, seminars, books, and other efforts. Armed with a good understanding of a plant, I can contribute to its increased popularity and trade. Companies who sell the plants I promote often benefit greatly from increased sales. Jerry Wu sent me an itinerary based on my list of requests. If horny goat continued to grow in the U.S. market, Jerry's company would benefit from increased demand. With a backpack filled with film and camera equipment, I boarded a jet in Boston and headed off to

Shanghai, on the southeastern coast of mainland China and the East China Sea.

What The Doctors Say

My jet touched down late at night at Pudong, a huge modern airport in the Shanghai countryside. Drenched in light, the sleek facility stood long and high, a glistening Great Wall. At baggage I was greeted by two men, Chen and Yu Yi, both of whom worked with Jerry Wu. I loaded my gear into their van, and we zoomed out into the dark Chinese night, for the forty-five minute ride into town. I liked Chen and Yu Yi right away. We struggled with little common language, but got on just fine nonetheless. They both seemed bright and good-humored. They'd make fine traveling companions.

The next morning I gazed out the window of my twentieth-floor hotel room. A bustling metropolis that was once a colonial city, Shanghai is becoming a forest of steel and glass. More than fifteen hundred skyscrapers were constructed in the last seven years. The skyline featured 20 percent of the world's construction cranes. The capitalist revolution in China is very well under way, with Shanghai at the epicenter of that thriving, energetic, unstoppable force. Western-style clothing is the norm, most major international banks have branch offices there, many U.S. corporations advertise on huge, high-tech billboards. The practice of herbal medicine and the herbal business are booming.

At the same time Shanghai is also a steamy tropical chaos, the law means little on the street. Even when a police officer stands in the middle of an intersection with a halt sign and a red light, traffic streams by unceasingly. Crossing the streets is a deadly proposition. Fortunately, the city has many tunnels and overpasses for pedestrians.

On my first evening in Shanghai, I gathered for dinner with six of Shanghai's top doctors of Traditional Chinese Medicine. The group included the chief physician of Shanghai's Longhua Hospital, a top gastroenterologist, a pharmacognosist, a plant chemist, and two other practicing medical doctors. The individuals at our table constituted a distinguished Chinese medical brain trust.

Medical doctor Diao Yuan Kuang explained the differences between TCM and western medicine. "Our tradition of practice is five thousand years old. We know from very good experience that TCM is highly effective. We successfully treat many difficult diseases, including rheumatoid arthritis, diabetes, and Parkinson's. In the United States, you have superior technology for diagnosis such as MRI, and we know that is effective as well. In TCM, we look at the whole person, while western physicians look at the disease. But the disease entity and the holistic picture are different. In the best of circumstances, the two will come together to create one dynamic medicine."

I asked about the role of herbs in TCM, to which Dr. Kuang responded, "Herbs are our primary medicines and can successfully treat most diseases. Not all, but most. They are the best and most effective medicines. And for promoting health, herbs and proper diet are superior." I asked if western doctors went to Shanghai to learn TCM. "We see over one hundred every month," answered Dr. Hu Jinhua, chief physician of Shanghai's Longhua Hospital and one of China's leading brain specialists.

I asked the question foremost on my mind. "What do you think about epimedium? Is it truly effective as a sex-enhancer?"

There were smiles all around, and the affirmative shaking of heads.

"Oh, yes, yes," exclaimed Doctor Kuang. "We have all used epimedium for decades in our practices. It is the very best sexual tonic for both men and women."

I probed further. Does the plant truly help with erectile function as some claim? Both Dr. Kuang and Dr. Xiao Tong Shen explained that in clinical practice, they have used epimedium to successfully treat erectile problems, to boost waning libido, and to rebuild youthful sexual vitality. "It gives you back your sexual strength," noted Dr. Kuang with emphasis.

I asked about restoring women's sexual desire during menopause, when libido often wanes. Dr. Kuang commented, "Women can regain their sexual desire when they take epimedium." According to Doctor Kuang, "it is a natural sexual tonic and does not interfere with natural hormonal balance. It is excellent for women." The others at the table explained that epimedium is used as the lead herb in a host of formulas for building sexual vitality and regenerating sexual vigor. In the estimation of some of China's greatest physicians, horny goat weed is the real thing. I had unequivocal confirmation of horny goat weed's sex-enhancing effects from the top docs in China.

The Road To Bozhou

When I told Jerry Wu that I wanted to see herb markets, he took that as a clear request to proceed directly to the largest herb market on earth. To get there required a van, two drivers, Jerry, and Chen, who as it turned out is Jerry's top man. I discovered that Chen got things done. When the van needed repair, Chen took care of it. In scouting restaurants, Chen was in charge. If a place passed the Chen test, we ate there. If it failed, we moved on. Chen was the fixer, an indispensable man to have on our side.

"We are going to the herb market in Bozhou, which will require a little travel," Jerry explained. To get there, we would drive from Shanghai on the coast of Jiangsu Province, to China's Central Plains region at the far northwestern corner of neighboring Anhui Province. The twelve-hour road trip from Shanghai was long, hot, and very bumpy. We crossed the majestic Yangtse River in Nanjing and rolled past endless emerald green rice paddies, small tea plantations, aquaculture ponds of mussels, gigantic lotus ponds, corn and squash fields, vegetable gardens, and lazy oxen and water buffalo. People by the thousands bent over in the fields in water up to their shins, planting rice, China's primary starch food.

As we approached the fertile plains of Bozhou, we saw fields of wheat, corn, soybeans, sorghum, sweet potato, tobacco, and medicinal herbs. The agriculturally diverse region is also home to large-scale cultivation of hot chiles, peaches, mulberries, rapeseed, apples, powlonia trees for timber, the largest walnut farm in Asia, and an astounding 600,000 acres of medicinal herbs! Our group was headed to the very center of that area's herbal commerce, in a city that was capital of the Shang Dynasty 3,700 years ago.

Little did we suspect that we were an official delegation. We pulled our van to the shoulder of the road on the outskirts of town, where city dignitaries received our small group with expressions of welcome and handshakes all around. A police escort with blaring sirens and flashing lights led our retinue across the picturesque Wohe River and into the city of Bozhou to a hotel frequented by Communist party bosses and officials. That evening at a sumptuous dinner of regional specialties with city officials, we were toasted with Bozhou's famous and surprisingly potent Gu Jing Gong Jiu liquor. Try saying that ten times fast after twelve cups. It cannot be done. What a welcome.

The World's Largest Herb Market

The next day I rode in a Chinese cop car whose suspension had long ago given out, as yet another siren-blaring police escort delivered us to the immense Bozhou herb market. Bozhou has a history of more than four hundred years in the commercial cultivation and trading of medicinal herbs, and the city is home to the annual Chinese national medicinal herbs fair. Of the four major herb markets in China, Bozhou is the largest. Occupying eighty-five acres, the market is home to more than six thousand traders who sell their healthful wares five days a week, at an annual sales volume of 20 billion yuan, about 250 million U.S. dollars. Buyers from China, Singapore, Malaysia, Japan, and Korea negotiate for tons of precious herbal products. Non-Asian visitors, especially a tall gringo holding a camera, are apparently rare. Upon our arrival, my companions and I drew a crowd that stayed with us the whole time.

No amount of prior explanation could have adequately prepared us for the grand scale of the market. The central market building, with 156,000 square meters of interior selling space, was jammed with thousands of people and thousands of herbal displays. Large jute and hemp sacks of loose herbs stood packed against each other from one end of the hall to the other. Truck-high displays of white and red ginsengs ran in rows. Shiny mystical reishi mushrooms, crenellated maitake, and worm-shaped wild cordyceps in high piles seemed to go on forever in the fungus section. In the animal and insect areas, neat stacks of pressed snakes, geckos, centipedes, and scorpions were startling in both their grand size and their carnal aroma. It was a vast, strange scene.

As we struggled through curious, pressing crowds, Jerry explained the use of various medicinal herbs, while big Chen kindly but firmly aided our progress by picking people up and setting them down out of our way. On both the upper and lower levels of the gigantic main hall, we found large displays of dried horny goat weed in cloth sacks. When dealers noticed our apparent interest in epimedium, they broke out in smiles. "Very good for sex," one told us. Another remarked, "That will make you sexually strong." The comments we received were universal. I inquired into the tonnage of horny goat weed that sold every year. Nobody knew for sure, but given that the herb plays a role in numerous popular formulas, traders said that the figure was high. Amid the awesome spectacle of the world's largest herb market, horny goat weed was declared the reigning champion of herbal sex-enhancers.

A number of herbal traders asked me what I was doing in the herb market. When I explained that I was investigating herbs in general and epimedium in particular, they smiled. "In the United States," I explained, "epimedium is now a very big product. You will sell a lot of it over the next few years," I predicted. The traders seemed enthusiastic about the prospect of Americans consuming horny goat weed.

Paying Respects to Hua Tuo

On the outskirts of Bozhou, we visited an ornate stone and tile temple to pay our respects to Hua Tuo, a great doctor of the

Eastern Han Dynasty. Born in Bozhou and regarded as one of the fathers of Traditional Chinese Medicine, Hua Tuo was expert in medical theory and practice. He developed the famous Five Animal Exercise system of longevity fitness and is credited with having invented surgery under anaesthesia. In the manner of traditional Taoist physicians, Hua Tuo was apparently a paragon of health and vitality, a keen scholar, and an astute observer of human nature. His manner of counseling patients is to this day the stuff of legend and the reverence his memory inspires borders on deification. Thanks to new friends, I had been taken into the very heart of China's precious health treasures.

Journey to the Source

Our stay in Bozhou included a tour of several hundred thousand hectares of medicinal plant cultivation. There, hundreds of varieties are cultivated to ensure a plentiful supply for the expanding Chinese and export markets. But due to its abundance in the wild epimedium was not among them. We loaded back into the van for another road trip. Our expanded group included a medicinal plant expert named Sheng, who would lead us to a major wild source of horny goat weed. Struggling down the road with a bad clutch, we headed in a southeasterly direction. Our destination was Tianmushan, a large mountain area in the northern corner of Zhejiang Province. After about eight hours of hard driving, we pulled into Nanjing for the night. The van went to a mechanic for repair, and we all caught a few hours of sleep—*after* an overly large midnight meal and endless rounds of beer toasts.

The next day as we journeyed to remote Tianmu Mountain,

Sheng explained the collection of epimedium. "All epimedium is picked wild, and this raises a lot of questions. The plant is very abundant. It grows all over, so there is a lot. But people ask about epimedium being overharvested. There is nothing to worry about in that regard. As long as the roots remain in the ground, it comes up every year. We only ever pick the leaves, never the roots. So epimedium is always there. And since nobody applies any chemicals to wild plants, it is clean and pure."

After a long drive on bad roads, we arrived at Tianmushan, where we cruised up the western slope of the mountain into tall stands of fragrant pine and huge, ancient ginkgo. Jerry pointed at the ginkgo trees. "Many experts say that the first ginkgo trees came from this very place." The brain-enhancing ginkgo trees stood tall and majestic, their distinctive green leaves fluttering in a mild breeze.

We parked at the end of the road, about two-thirds of the way up Tianmu. With Sheng in the lead, we hiked off into dense forest and up a rugged trail on the mountain's steep western peak. The tropical sun beat down on us when we stepped out of the woods, and we were drenched in sweat as we made our way up the mountain. "Most of the epimedium on the mountain has already been picked this year," Sheng informed us. "But further up near the peak we will find plenty. The pickers don't like to climb that high." We came to a rock outcropping, where we saw our first clusters of epimedium growing in the wild. "The plant likes rocks," Shen told us.

From that point on toward the peak we found numerous clusters of epimedium that had escaped the attention of pickers who had collected the plant only a month before. We stopped repeatedly on the steep slope to admire spectacular views of the mountainous countryside. Vistas of forests and lakes and picturesque hillsides stretched for more than fifty miles. Chen laughed. "Well, we found the weed." And it was true. We came, we climbed, and we found horny goat weed.

Back down the mountainside after our hot climb, we shed our shirts at a chilly stream and soaked ourselves before returning to the road. After several hours of driving, we had a late dinner in the city of Hangzhou, and toasted our success with a potent liquor made of rice alcohol, cobra snake, wild ginseng, and wolfberry. Ours was a happy group, filled with the enthusiasm that comes from a mission fulfilled.

Herbal Alchemy

One of the major challenges of botanical medicine is how to translate herbal remedies that work in the field into effective products on store shelves. This is where extraction comes in. In Shanghai at the Draco manufacturing facility, Jerry Wu explained some of their process to us. "Traditional Chinese Medicine is primarily a teapot medicine. All different herbs are boiled in a teapot, and you drink the concentrated herbal tea when it is done. So we have figured out a system to make full-spectrum herbal extracts using only water extraction. In this way, we maintain the integrity of the plants, and we prepare them in a manner similar to the traditional method." Then he showed us a huge warehouse of botanicals ready for extraction, including about twenty tons of horny goat weed.

Processing at Draco is anything but traditional. Huge extraction vessels contain tons of herbs undergoing hot water extraction at high pressure—a far cry from a home teapot. The system is ingenious, and much of the equipment was custom designed by Jerry and his team. "We have certain equipment that was made just for us," he explained. After extraction, the concentrated fluid botanicals undergo spray drying, by a proprietary process, with no additives of any kind. "In this way, we get the most pure extract possible, and it is totally water soluble." I asked how much extract his company manufactures per month. "Right now we make 35 metric tons of extract per month, but we will be increasing that amount."

Draco employs highly trained lab technicians and maintains sophisticated laboratories with the latest analytical instruments, including Thin Layer Chromatography and High Performance Liquid Chromatography. The blending of science with tradition is an alchemical formula for success. "We are experiencing a great deal of demand for our pure herbal extracts," Jerry said. "People want traditional Chinese herbs, because they are highly effective. This is a very good time."

The End of the Trail

After a jam-packed tour in China, I had the goods. Our team had met with top docs, visited the largest herb market in the world, climbed Tianmu Mountain to the source of horny goat weed, and seen the processing of the plant into a stable, potent extract form. All the people we met endorsed horny goat weed without reservation. We had followed the plant from field to finished extract, and we came away profoundly impressed. Laden with field notes, bags of film to develop, and a few bottles of Bozhou's famous Gu Jing Gong Jiu liquor, I said goodbye to my new friends, boarded a jet and headed home.

The Erection Test

All the herbal market visits in the world don't mean that a product really works. Well, does it? In order to know that the Horny Goat Weed formula actually enhances sexual function, the product was submitted to New York's Dr. Steven Lamm for a human clinical study. The one study became two, and results were promising.

The first study conducted by Dr. Lamm was entitled, "The Effect of Pinnacle Horny Goat Weed on Sexual Satisfaction in Healthy Men and Men Treated with Viagra." In this trial, twenty-five healthy men and thirteen men who used Viagra were assigned to receive daily doses for forty-five days of two capsules (808 mg each capsule) of Pinnacle Horny Goat Weed formula. An additional four capsules were taken one to two hours prior to sexual activity to determine any effects on sexual interest, sexual performance, and overall sexual satisfaction. After forty-five days the study became double blind. This means that neither the patients nor the doctor knew who was getting the Horny Goat Weed formula and who were getting a placebo. This part of the trial included only those men (twenty healthy men and thirteen men on Viagra) who had reported a positive response in the first part of the trial.

All subjects were evaluated after the first forty-five days of treatment and finally after sixty days. Daily use of the Horny Goat Weed formula for a minimum of forty-five days resulted in enhanced sexual satisfaction in 60 percent of healthy men and in 45 percent of Viagra users. This is a good result overall, showing benefits from the herbal formula.

The second study conducted by Dr. Lamm was entitled, "The Effect of Pinnacle Horny Goat Weed on Penile Axial

Rigidity in Sexually Active Males." Basically, this study looked into exactly how hard an erection might result from using the herbal formula. In the study, fourteen sexually active men, ages twenty-five to fifty-five years old, took self-administered measurements of penile rigidity (hardness of erections), using a digital inflection rigidometer (DIR) soon after commencing sexual activity. They were then instructed to stop sexual activity. Approximately one hour after ingesting a dose of three capsules (808 mg each capsule) of the Horny Goat Weed formula, they resumed sexual activity and took additional measurements of penile rigidity to determine the effect of the product.

Of the eleven men who successfully completed the study, seven experienced increased penile rigidity as a result of using the herbal formula. Six men went from an adequate level of penile rigidity to a superior level of penile rigidity. One man who already had superior rigidity experienced an increase as well. The four men in this study who did not experience improved firmness of erections all found that they maintained an erection more easily. In other words, the Horny Goat Weed formula made most participants harder and enabled them all to keep an erection longer.

It appears that the popular Horny Goat Weed formula by Pinnacle improves erectile function. The formula contains a significant amount of MacaPure standardized maca (*Lepidium meyenii*) extract, which is discussed in the chapter on maca, High Plains Aphrodisiac, on page 145.

In Traditional Chinese Medicine, herbs are not typically used singly. They are virtually always taken in a formula. Strictly speaking, it is impossible to determine from the two studies conducted by Dr. Lamm whether the epimedium in Horny Goat Weed formula, or a synergy of all the ingredients, makes a difference. We do know though that this product delivers results—with few potential side effects—to those who wish to improve sexual function naturally, without the aid of pharmaceuticals.

The use of Horny Goat Weed formula among women is exceedingly popular. With women there are no turgidity tests. Women have given a surprising amount of unsolicited feedback to the manufacturer. Repeated use of the Horny Goat Weed formula significantly boosts female libido. The exact means by which this occurs is not known with certainty, but it is most likely due to the androgen-like activity of the epimedium, in conjunction with other botanicals in the formula. Men may have erectile function studies to back up anecdotal evidence, but women too have reported definite increases in libido.

Using Horny Goat Weed

Since there is clinical evidence demonstrating the efficacy of a particular product, I would recommend using the Pinnacle Horny Goat Weed formula. Follow the directions for use on the label, adjusting upward if you feel that you need more. See the resources section.

THE GODS MAKE LOVE

Ashwagandha

IN INDIA'S HINDU COSMOLOGY, THE GODS ARE FAR LESS stuffy than the Judeo-Christian God. They aren't robed ascetics with flowing gray beards, storming about amid ponderous clouds. Consider Lord Krishna, for example. This beautiful, androgenous blue god with wet eyes and pouty lips made headlines in the divine scriptures by making love to ten thousand voluptuous milkmaids in one amazing, priapic night. Lord Krishna seduced more women than Valentino and Cassanova combined and still managed to be completely at one with all the universe, manifest and unmanifest—past, present, and future.

Lord Siva, the mightiest of all the Hindu gods, is one lusty divinity, and has been depicted engaged in lewd naked dancing, his long hair erect. Lord Siva is known to dally and sport with lovely young maidens. He gives brilliant discourse on holy scripture while his eternal goddess counterpart Parvati sits in his lap, her silken skirt hiked up, her yoni firmly planted upon Lord Siva's divine root in the yab yum lovemaking position. Siva's symbol? A lingam, a stone phallus. The idea of divine discourse combined with heavenly intercourse is far more appealing than pulpit pounding scripture and a hard church pew. Plus, in moments of orgasm induced ecstasy, don't many people call out, "Oh God, oh God?" The ecstasies of sex and divine revelation are described in notably similar ways. Sex and the divine are a seemless fit.

Perhaps no other country enjoys such a long and colorful history of erotic exposition and ecstatic practices as India. The *Kama Sutra,* certainly the best known of all the love texts, originated in India. It details the many and varied ways to make love, from kissing to scratching, biting, fondling, caressing, and engaging in any and all manner of erotic and sexual actvities. The best-known aspects of the *Kama Sutra* are the diverse lovemaking positions, which combine sizzling eroticism with yogic flexibility and vivid imagination. The *Kama Sutra* is not the only exposition on the arts of love. A great many temples boast absolutely staggering works of erotic art, especially sculptures. Among the few hundred Indian temples I have visited, the most memorable is the Hoysala temple, which boasts over thirty thousand extravagant sandstone sculptures, many of which depict the gods making lusty, ecstatic love.

And then there is the profound science of yoga, which I have practiced on a daily basis for almost thirty-five years. Yoga is a deep well of spiritual practices and an enlivening system of methods, which switch on the sensitivity of the senses and liberate potent erotic energy. Not only does yoga practice imbue people with keen vitality, but many of the yoga postures themselves are in fact lovemaking positions. Yoga practice turns on the erotic flow within men and women as surely as it awakens the mind to a greater consciousness. It does so by stimulating nerves and glands, improving the balance of hormones within the body, and infusing the entire system with a higher level of energy. Yoga and sex are inextricably linked in a web of pleasure and ecstatic fulfillment.

Part of traditional yoga practice is the study of medicinal plants, as many yoga scriptures attest. In India, yogis are often experts in the preparation and use of medicinal plants. Of all the vitality-enhancing, sex-boosting, erotic-awakening plants in the entire Indian yogic pharmacopoeia, none is as revered for its benefits and profound in its effects as ashwagandha. In India, ashwagandha is the aphrodisiac that has no equal.

Medicine of the Gods

At the Government Ayurvedic Research Center in Bangalore, India, I observed a scene from medieval times. Before me in a dimly lit stone basement, four men clad only in dhotis and turbans managed the cooking of an herbal formula in an immense cauldron that rested on massive stone blocks over an open, roaring fire. The room baked like an oven. The cauldron was of sufficiently large size to contain two adults standing. Employing stirring paddles the size and shape of boat oars, the sweating men took turns stirring the sweet-smelling mixture inside the cauldron. Turbans askew, they strained slender backs and bandy arms under the intense labor. Dr. Prabakhan, an Ayurvedic specialist, explained that the formula being made would be cooled and bottled, and then shipped to clinics. A principle ingredient in the mixture was ashwagandha, *Withania somnifera*. The most widely used of all plants in India's millennia-old system of Ayurveda, ashwagandha is also that country's most widely used hot plant, for ashwagandha enhances sex as surely as fire heats a pot.

"We make herbal medicines for over fifty clinics here," explained Dr. Prabakhan. "We send them entirely free, and people go to the clinics and receive these medicines at no cost. This way, we can help to meet the health needs of many people who cannot afford to pay for medicines, as they are very poor." I admired the approach to health care he described, wishing that in the United States health care were based more on people's needs, instead of on profitability, shareholder stock value, and patent law.

After roasting in the infernally hot basement, we walked upstairs to a cavernous hall where herbs were stored prior to their use in medicines dispensed to many Indians as a free service. In the hall, groaning sacks of herbs smelled woody, sweet, and aromatic in a hundred different ways. "Where is the ashwagandha?" I asked Dr. Prabakhan. He led me to an area where dozens of large sacks lay piled one on top of another. The sacks were loosely closed, and I could see that they contained pieces of dried root. It was like looking at stacks of gold. For ashwagandha serves the body's needs in many beneficial ways.

Ayurveda, the oldest known system of health care in the world today, is derived from the first-known inhabitants of the Indian subcontinent, the Dravidians; from the Aryan culture; and from the Mughul Empire. The traditions of these three cultures combined to form a comprehensive system of diagnosis, prescription, and treatment that blends diet, herbs, minerals, meditation, exercise, and various physical therapies. The ancient traditional principles and practices of Ayurveda are being corroborated by modern scientists in disciplines ranging from advanced forms of diagnosis to pharmacy. How the ancients figured out what they did, in such a comprehensive way, remains a profound mystery.

According to the principles of Ayurveda, each person is composed of a unique balance of three primary forces, which interact on physical, psychological, and spiritual levels. These forces, known as *doshas,* are named *vatta, pitta,* and *kapha.* *Vatta* is made up of the elements air and space, and is responsible for all motion and energy flow within the body. When *vatta* is imbalanced, the result may be constipation, menstrual problems, poor digestion, and a restless or anxious mind. *Pitta* is made up of fire and water, and is responsible for metabolism, digestion, and energy production. When *pitta* is out of balance, one can become angry, digestion may suffer, and skin eruptions and ulcers may result. *Kapha,* made of earth and water, is responsible for the structure of the body. When *kapha* is out of balance energy diminishes, enthusiasm wanes, and colds, flu, congestion, and excess often result. According to Ayurveda, disequilibrium among the three *doshas* results in diseases of various kinds.

In Ayurveda, a patient is diagnosed not just according to the disease he or she may exhibit, but according to the condition of the *doshas.* Each person is typically dominant in one *dosha.* Thus, a *kapha* dominant patient with a cold and a *pitta* patient with a cold would be treated differently. In order to restore proper balance of the *doshas* to rebuild health, an Ayurvedic treatment plan is tailored to the individual, and incorporates proper diet, exercise, meditation, the use of specific medicinal herbal formulas, and any of several cleansing methods designed to rid the body of toxins. Health, according to this system, is not merely the absence of disease, but a dynamic state of harmony. In this state of harmony, inner metabolic fire is strong, energy is abundant, and the mind is at peace. Ayurvedic philosophy is brilliantly summed up in the following phrase from an ancient text: "May all be happy, may all be healthy, may all experience that which is good, and let no one suffer."

In fact, Ayurveda does have its own patron god, Dhanwantari. A manifestation of the god Vishnu, Dhanwantari has as his mission to enhance humanity's awareness of holy truth in the world. It's a big job that requires four arms. In one hand, Dhanwantari holds a leach for bloodletting to facilitate recovery from disease. A second hand holds a pot containing a precious elixir of longevity. A third hand carries a conch shell, which the god uses to blow the sound of *om,* the sound of all creation. And in his fourth hand Dhanwantari holds a chakra, a spinning vortex of energy, which destroys ignorance and darkness. Dhanwantari's vehicle of service in the world is the divine medical system of Ayurveda, which eliminates impediments in body and mind to health and spiritual realization, the true purpose of life. Everywhere you travel in India, anywhere that Ayurveda is practiced or its products sold, you will see a likeness of the patron god Dhanwantari. It may be a simple drawing, a beautiful painting, a marble statue, or a crude carving out of wood, but it will be there.

The Great Hot Plant

Of all the medicinal plants used in India's several-millennia-old tradition of Ayurveda, ashwagandha, *Withania somnifera,* is the most highly prized. Use of the root can be traced back as far as 3,000 years. Ashwagandha is classified as a *rasayan,* a rejuvenating or life-extending agent. The *rasayan* are the most esteemed of Ayurveda's herbs, as they imbue the user with life itself. The root of the plant appears in remedies for cough, rheumatism, gynecological disorders, fatigue, emaciation, inflammation, ulcers, sore eyes, and diminished brain function.

Ashwagandha is also India's most potent hot plant. It is used equally by men and women, and is widely prescribed by physicians to adults with low libido, and to improve sexual function. In the system of Ayurvedic medicine, ashwagandha is the penultimate plant. I was in southern India to research the plant, and to learn about its potent, sex-enhancing properties.

The Human Garden

After my foray to the Government Ayurvedic Research Center, I met up with Dr. S. K. Mitra and Dr. Rangesh Paramesh, both executives at Himalaya Drug Company, India's largest and most modern maker of herbal medicines for health. I had made contact with them prior to my trip, and they had generously agreed to assist me in my research efforts. The two showed up for our meeting in impeccable suits. I wore shorts and a short-sleeved shirt, which seemed more suitable to the broiling temperature, which hovered around 36° C (96° F).

As we sped across Bangalore under a sweltering sun, Dr. Mitra described the current popularity of Ayurveda. "Ayurveda has always been important to Indian culture. It goes back thousands of years. But now, thanks to international interest in plant medicine, Ayurveda is even more popular. This is good and bad. It is good, because it leads people away from harsh and potentially dangerous drugs. But it is also a problem, because there is a demand for much, much more herbal material. Now, big movie stars promote their interest in Ayurveda, so even the young people are interested." Mitra shook his head.

"For a long time, you could get all the plants you need from the hills and natural areas. But all that has changed. Today we must cultivate plants to meet demand."

A roiling spume of fine brown dust behind us, we pulled up to the Dhanvantari Vana Ayurvedic Herbal Garden. Featuring over five hundred species of medicinal plants, the garden is a joint project between the University of Bangalore and the Indian government. From aloe to ashwagandha, the one-hundred-acre garden displayed thousands of seedlings and cuttings of each plant. "You see," Dr. Paramesh explained, "here farmers can come and get seedlings, which they can plant on their own land. When the plants are ready for harvest, the farmers can make more money than growing rice or collecting green coconuts. Plus, growing medicinal plants is essential now if Ayurveda is to continue to thrive and prosper." Knowing that I wanted to see ashwagandha, the two doctors led me to a large section of the garden where several thousand small ashwagandha plants were ready for replanting.

"The reason there is so much ashwagandha here is that it is the very number-one, most-popular plant in all of India," Dr. Mitra told me. "A great many formulas in Ayurveda use ashwagandha." I asked about the sexual effects of the plant. "For that purpose it is the best of the best. Men and women take ashwagandha to rebuild sexual vitality and to restore proper and healthy sexual function. All doctors recommend it. It is the supreme medicinal plant." Does Himalaya Drug offer sex tonics containing ashwagandha? "Yes, of course," Dr. Mitra assured me with a smile.

In the middle of the Dhanvantari Vana Ayurvedic Herbal Garden, we found a garden about one quarter acre in size, in the shape of a human body. The outline of the body was detailed in stones. At each part of the body, various medicinal plants grew which addressed the needs of that bodily area. Digestive herbs grew in the region of the stomach and bowels. Herbs for the brain grew at the head. Anti-inflammatory herbs grew at the joints. All the herbs were labeled for easy identification. The human garden was an excellent and clever idea, and a marvelous teaching tool. In the genital region, several healthy specimens of ashwagandha grew, lush and green. India always surprises me, and the human garden was exemplary of the kind of ingenuity I have encountered repeatedly in that most remarkable country.

The Plant in the Ground

Muhammed Majeed loves his family and honors them by naming businesses for each member. His large and highly successful botanical extraction company in India is called Sami, named after his eldest daughter. His U.S.-based sales and distribution company for Ayurvedic extracts, called Sabinsa, is named after his wife. Not to be content with only two thriving businesses, Muhammed also operates Anju, a European Ayurvedic herbal distribution business named after his younger daughter. I wondered to myself if Muhammed Majeed would feel obliged to start a new corporation if his wife gave birth to another child? And what if triplets arrived?

Sitting in the expansive shaded gardens of Bangalore's Taj West End Hotel, the grit and dust of India seemed a world away. Muhammed and I faced a table of skewers of chicken, grilled vegetables, rice, and several regional dishes. We drank chilled lemonade and discussed the herbal trade, especially ashwagandha. In the United States, Majeed's company Sabinsa is the largest supplier of ashwagandha extract. In India, he and his employees devote a lot of time and energy to securing an adequate supply of the plant. "You see, there is a lot of pressure to secure this plant. The demand is quite intense. We are working on this problem."

By arrangement of Muhammed Majeed, the next morning I found myself at SAMI's experimental farm outside of Bangalore, in the company of herbal expert Suresh Kumar and agronomist Anil Chojar, who worked for the USDA for many years. We surveyed a field of rich brown soil, where shirtless barefoot laborers swung heavy picks through the air as they broke up the soil for planting. The air baked like a furnace. In that environment, only strong plants can survive, and we looked closely at some ashwagandha that appeared to be thriving in the unforgiving swelter. The name *ashwagandha* derives from the ancient Sanskrit language and means "smells like a horse," which it does if you get close and take a good whiff.

I found the plant pleasing to look at. A small woody shrub, ashwagandha features elliptical green leaves, small uniform five-petaled flowers, and red seeds. The plant flowers year-round, but the root of the plant is the prize, which Anil Chojar showed me by having one of the SAMI farm workers hack a plant out of the ground. A long taproot and a mass of smaller roots held clumps of soil. According to the American Herbal Pharmacopoeia, an acre of cultivated ashwagandha will yield about 225 kilos of root, which when dry reduces to around 70 kilos. It takes a year to bring the plant to maturity. Harvest is usually between January and March. The plant is forgiving, too, and requires little attention and no irrigation, even in the parched climate of southern India. Ashwagandha is a strong and vigorous plant, thriving where other plants wither and die.

Consider the fact that India requires thousands of tons of ashwagandha each year to make various Ayurvedic preparations, and you get a vivid sense of the need for gigantic-scale cultivation. One ton of dried root would require approximately thirteen acres of the plant under cultivation. One thousand tons would require thirteen thousand acres. Suresh Kumar explained that SAMI hoped to build up a substantial ashwagandha cultivation enterprise to become less dependent on other sources over time. Large-scale cultivation of ashwagandha had been ongoing for many years in both Rajasthan and Madhya Pradesh states, but still demand continued to exert tremendous pressure on supply. Wild supplies were being overharvested, especially where most abundant in warmer regions.

The Road To Ooti

To learn more about India's medicinal plants, especially ashwagandha, I chose to travel to south India's Nilgiri Hills, to the JSS College of Pharmacy. That school is a major center of scientific inquiry into Ayurveda's medicinal plants. Traveling south in a white Tata Sumo, I chatted with H. Prakash, a secretary on loan from Muhammed. Thirty-two years old, married, punctual, courteous and observant, Prakash was educated as a lawyer. At the wheel, twenty-one-year-old Prasad drove with testosterone and the horn. Unkempt, somewhat disheveled, and highly affable, Prasad contributed admirably to the pandemonium of India's chaotic traffic.

The road hosted a riot of trucks, buses, cars, vans, bicycles, scooters, motorcycles, scooter taxis, oxcarts, tractors, cows, dogs, wandering ascetics, sari-clad women, children playing, horns blaring, diesel smoke spewing, drivers waving and shouting, and bicycles laden with impossibly huge loads of water coconuts. Women balanced large parcels on their heads. Trucks passed buses passing cars, all careening through the Indian countryside. The fronts of "Public carriers" were festooned with glitter, holy decals, and statues of deities. These large, ornately decorated trucks carry any type of goods anywhere, and are ubiquitous throughout India. Pedestrians fled across the road as gaps opened and closed. Everybody cut everybody else off. Nobody displayed any courtesy of any kind. Horns blared. Trucks groaned under unimaginable loads.

We rode long hard hours and eventually began to approach the Nilgiri Hills from the north. We went up in elevation and drove through part of Bandipur wildlife refuge. There we passed a dozen or more wild forest elephants, great strong animals with powerful bodies and nut brown hides. We admired the elephants from a safe distance. Riding through the forest, we also observed deer, peacocks, and monkeys of all sizes.

Eventually we made our destination. Ootacamund, referred to most widely as Ooty, offered refreshing air, a profusion of garden flowers in bloom, and the indelible stamp of former British colonial rule. English cottages with slat shutters and gingerbread trim were surrounded by neatly tended grounds. The place displayed a Raj-era charm. We pulled up to the Savoy, a former British school turned lodging, surrounded by beautiful gardens, trimmed and shaped hedges, and manicured lawns.

After a night's sleep I headed across town to meet two top plant experts, Dr. B. Suresh, Principal and Professor of Pharmacology at JSS College, and Dr. Subbaraju, the school's head of pharmacognosy. We walked through the college gardens, which featured numerous plants employed in Ayurveda. Later in Suresh's office, we talked about ashwagandha. "It is certainly most widely used," Suresh told me. "Ashwagandha is used in many cases, for virtually every condition. It is also especially good for restoring vitality and full sexual potency. We work with many clinicians, and we get very good information about the results they obtain with patients. Ashwagandha is not a myth as far as its sexual effects are concerned. The root is very potent, and it unquestionably builds sexual vitality."

I asked both Suresh and Subbaraju about the traditional use of ashwagandha among hill tribes. In the Nilgiri Hills, five distinct tribal groups dwell in the forests. Subbaraju has studied these tribal people and has extensively documented their medicines. He is the definitive scientific expert on hill tribe medicines. "Among the tribals, ashawagandha is also used for sexual purposes. This use is so effective, the tribal people, whose medicine is different from traditional Ayurveda, still use ashwagandha for sex. You can ask any of the tribals what ashwagandha is for, and sex will be one of the very first uses they describe." Two of India's most learned and scientifically astute experts in medicinal plants agreed that ashwagandha is superior to virtually all other plants in the Ayurvedic pharmacopoeia.

"I will take you to see beautiful ashwagandha in the Eastern Ghats," Subbaraju promised. "There you will see some very amazing specimens, very large and large roots." He looked proud and delighted to share ashwagandha with me.

Ashwagandha's Chemical Soul

JSS College of Pharmacy boasts several modern laboratories where students and senior researchers investigate the phytochemicals—the natural plant compounds—in many medicinal plants. Researchers at JSS and other centers of plant research have discovered numerous compounds in ashwagandha. The plant is rich in potent alkaloids, among which are withamosine, visamine, cuscohygrine, anahygrine, tropine, pseudotropine, anaferine, isopelletierine, and withaferin A. The plant contains novel compounds known as withanolides, which are typically used to standardize the potency of extracts. Whether one or two of these compounds are responsible for the plant's health benefits, or whether ashwagandha's power derives from a complex synergy of all its natural constituents, is a matter which may take a long time to solve by scientific means. One of the lab heads at JSS showed me some notes about components from ashwagandha. "We work very hard to understand the plants, to know what is inside them. Then we can figure out what these compounds do in a living system and advance the science of plant medicine." According to research conducted at JSS and elsewhere, components in ashwagandha possess tonic, antiinflammatory, aphrodisiac, immunity-enhancing, anxiety-relieving, and nerve-sedative properties.

Animal and Human Studies

I would like to be able to say that many human studies show that ashwagandha is a superior sex enhancer, but there are no clinical studies on this use of ashwagandha. But the root enjoys three thousand years of such an application, by millions of satisfied people. While no clinical studies on the aphrodisiac effects of ashwagandha have been conducted to date, legions of people have gotten such an effect. This is in fact far more significant. In India, studying ashwagandha to see if the root demonstrates aphrodisiac properties would be like conducting a study to see if people get wet when they take showers. These effects are self-evident, reinforced by millennia of results.

The Indian *Materia Medica* recommends use of ashwagandha for general debility, impotence, general aphrodisiac purposes, brain fatigue, low sperm count, nervous exhaustion, and in any cases in which general vigor must be restored. For men and women, for the old and the young, ashwagandha builds strength from within. Often, this strength and vitality manifests as newfound or restored sexual vigor and function. One Ayurvedic aphrodisiac formula combines one part ashwagandha to ten parts milk and one part ghee (clarified butter). You boil the mixture down until only ghee remains. This end product is called Ashwagandha Ghrita. You take about a heaping tablespoon of this mixture in the morning and in the evening, and according to ancient texts, you will experience a significant boost in libido and sexual stamina.

Ashwagandha has been studied as an adaptogen, that class of natural plant agents that enhance overall immunity and build nonspecific resistance to various stresses. In one human clinical study, ashwagandha improved overall mental aptitude and reaction time.

In animal studies, ashwagandha demonstrates significant stress-fighting power. This is unquestionably key to the plant's sex-enhancing powers. Stress factors of all kinds compromise virtually every system of the body, producing deleterious chemicals caused by stress, which in turn diminish the function of organs and glands. In the domino effect of the ravages of stress on the human system, fatigue, reduced immunity, and sexual debility go hand in hand. The overwhelming stresses of life leave people feeling devitalized. When you take ashwagandha, that equation begins to turn around. As an adaptogen, the root helps the body to normalize all aspects of healthy function. One of the many noticeable areas in which this turn-around takes place is sexual. Men and women who have lost their desire for sex or have lost function, find that they become aroused again—and ready to engage in sexual activity.

Cobras in the Cane

In the company of the ever faithful Prakash and Prasad, Dr. Subburaju and I headed from the cool Nilgiri Hills down to the broiling plains of the Eastern Ghats. "This way you can see for yourself some very large ashwagandha that is planted there," he told me. As we sped along in the arid and dusty heat, Subburaju pointed out numerous medicinal plants. All along the way, we saw neem trees, the leaves of which are used in soaps and toiletries and which also yield natural insecticides. We stopped to admire some datura, whose compounds are used in modern medicine, one of which, scopolamine, is dropped into the eyes to dilate pupils for opthalmic exams.

After hours of driving, we came to a small village surrounded by a great many fields of sugarcane. Subburaju led me to a blue house and introduced me to the head of the house, a Mr. Barhi. We sat and drank cool lemonade before heading to a growing area. Subburaju explained to me: "You see, these people are growing ashwagandha. I think that it will be a very good crop for them. You will observe for yourself, even in this heat the plants are very healthy." We eventually came to a large garden area where various vegetables were planted. Nearby was a plot with many large, healthy ashwagandha. The plants were appreciably bigger than the others I had seen near Bangalore, and I remarked at that. "Yes," Subbaraju agreed, "the soil conditions are very good here. If the market demand is going to be met, then people here can grow a great deal of ashwagandha. As much as they can grow, the market will take it."

Barhi and another man used a pick to dig out one large plant to show us the root. The plant did not yield easily, but the two men attacked the soil with determination, and in a few minutes the root was theirs. I cut a small piece with my pocket knife and chewed it. The taste was pleasant enough. The men smiled at my appreciation and gave the root to Subbaraju and me to take back to Ooty. I asked if the people in the village intended to grow a lot more ashwagandha. Yes, Barhi told me. It will be a good crop, and the money for the root will be better than the money for many other plants.

Back at Barhi's house, I asked why the beds were suspended from ropes attached to the ceiling, instead of standing on legs. Barhi smiled. "The cane fields are full of cobras. At night, they slither all around, and sometimes they make their way into the house. Hanging the beds affords a little protection." Later, when Subbaraju and I began the long journey back, I took a long look at the glistening fields of cane, and my mind was filled with thoughts of snakes making their silent way through the local households in the dead of night.

The Doctor's Prescription

Days later I found myself in Trivandrum, in Kerala state, where Ayurveda originated. I was there to meet Dr. Shetey, a specialist in reproductive and sexual health. Dr. Shetey ran her own clinic and pharmacy, and all visible evidence suggested that she enjoyed a busy practice. Her waiting room was full, and her pharmacy had a steady stream of people going in and out.

Nonetheless, Dr. Shetey took time from her busy schedule to meet and talk with me.

"Do you see both men and women?"

"Yes, in my practice I see men and women. The women come to me for all their gynecological and obstetric needs. So I see women of all ages, for checkups and also when they are pregnant or in poor health. With the men it is different. I mostly see them when they are having sexual difficulties, either a loss of libido or some impairment in erectile function." I asked Dr. Shetey what she thought of Ayurveda for sexual health. She smiled in a knowing manner. "There is no medicine at our disposal that will do for sexual health what ashwagandha will do. It is a plant that can be used in all conditions, without concern for negative effects. With women, I give ashwagandha as a matter of course when they have experienced a drop in libido, usually due to the onset of menopause. But with men, I give it to them not only for low libido, but when they are having problems with impotence."

I asked Dr. Shetey to tell me about the efficacy of ashwagandha. "It is absolutely the very best possible thing to rebuild sexual health. I have seen women who did not have any desire at all, and when they use ashwagandha, they become quite amorous again. It almost uniformly brings back full sexual vitality. With men, there is not only the issue of desire, which ashwagandha restores quickly. But also many men are devastated when they cannot achieve an erection. In many cases, the use of ashwagandha restores them back to healthy function. I have seen hundreds of impotent men regain their sexual ability. It is like bringing them back from the dead. And also then there is the benefit, not only of achieving a healthy erection once again, but also a great improvement in self-esteem." I asked if

Dr. Shetey would recommend ashwagandha to anyone suffering from low libido or impotence. "Absolutely. Ashwagandha imbues people with great vitality. It makes you very strong from within. For the purposes of sexual health, it is the greatest of all medicines."

Using Ashwagandha

A variety of ashwagandha products have made their way into the U.S. supplement market. If you are going to use the powdered root, then the *Ayurvedic Pharmacopoeia of India* recommends 3–6 grams daily.

Most people will prefer a tableted or encapsulated product. Some companies now offer extracts of ashwagandha, standardized to a specified level of withanolides. A daily dose is approximately 250–500 milligrams of extract standardized to 4–5 percent withanolides. See the resource section for recommended brands.

HOT AND DAMP PLACES

Catuaba

"YOU KNOW WHAT IS THE SAYING ABOUT CATUABA, BIG GUY?"
I eyed Bernie sideways and shook my head. "They say that until
a man reaches age sixty, the child belongs to him. After that, the
son is catuaba's!" Bernie gave a wide smile. "So what that means
is that as you age, if you gonna get a woman pregnant, then after a certain point it is because the catuaba keeps you sexually
potent." I smiled and gazed out the window of our jet as we descended through muscular clouds of steely gray to a view of the
vast expanse of the Brazilian Amazon rain forest and the largest
river on earth. There in the forest, Bernie and I would research
the Amazon's most famous sex enhancing plant, catuaba.

My friend and traveling companion, Bernie Peixoto was born
and raised in the Brazilian Amazon. An Eur-eu-wa-wa Indian,
his tribal name is Ipupiara, which means fresh water dolphin.
Bernie bridges a number of cultures at once. Under the auspices
of native elders, he spent years training to become a shaman,
one who travels back and forth freely between the phenomenal
and spirit worlds. As an Amazonian shaman, Bernie performs
healings, leads vision quests, and seeks information from the

spirit realm. He's easy to find on the World Wide Web now, with a search for "Ipupiara." Bernie has traveled far from his original village in the rain forest to the modern world, bridging cultures and sharing traditional knowledge.

Bernie also applied his keen mind to academics as well and earned a Ph.D. in anthropology. In that role, Bernie is a peerless expert in the people and culture of the Amazon and possesses vast knowledge of indigenous peoples from the Pacific Peruvian coast to Belem, Brazil, where the Amazon river rushes into the Atlantic Ocean. He lives with his wife in Washington, D.C., has worked as an adviser to the Smithsonian Institute, and counts Chelsea Clinton as one of his many students. Bernie's broad knowledge of the environment and cultures of the northern Amazon, combined with his command of over ten languages, made him not only a brilliantly informed companion, but an ideal guide.

Herbalist of the Upper Amazon

The hot, steaming northern Brazilian city of Manaus lies at the intersection of the great Amazon River and the massive Rio Negro, whose waters naturally run coffee black. Bernie and I hailed a battered Datsun taxi, whose driver threaded us through narrow, crowded streets to the Mercado Antonio Lisboa, the municipal market. A century-old cast-iron structure at the Manaus waterfront, the once splendid Mercado was fashioned after Les Halles in Paris. Today, the bustling Mercado is faded and old, its formerly gleaming marble counters dulled and stained with the blood of one hundred years of butchered fish and meat.

The Mercado along with the ornate Manaus Opera House stand as vestiges of the opulent age of the Amazon rubber boom from the late 1800s to the 1920s. Latex from rubber trees in the surrounding rain forest supplied a hungry world rubber market, and gold flowed in the streets. The cosmopolitan jewel of the Amazon, Manaus became a city of refined culture and high society. Eventually the Amazon rubber industry crashed beyond salvation when Indonesian plantations began to produce a greater volume of rubber more quickly and cheaply. The French bakers, Italian stonemasons, Viennese musicians, and glitterati of Manaus society departed. Today Manaus is a crowded and diverse tropical city of tribal, Portuguese, Chinese, and other people. Situated in the middle of the largest rain forest on earth, the city of Manaus teems with life. The entire Manuas waterfront and river region runs heavy with boat traffic day and night. Riverside stilt shacks by the hundreds perch precariously against the muddy hills of the city's riversides. On the river, large gas barges refill the tanks of thousands of river-going vessels large and small.

Bernie and I had journeyed to the Brazilian Amazon to conduct research on catuaba, *Erythroxylum catuaba*, the Amazon's most widely used hot plant. Our journey would take us from Manaus into the rain forest with native guides. Our first stop was to see Antonio Matas, the best-known herbal healer in Manaus, and the Amazon's most widely filmed and interviewed herbal expert. His popularity owes in no small part to the fact that Antonio runs a large herbal shop in the very center of the Mercado, the most visited spot in that Amazonian city. Television producers make a beeline to the Mercado, where Antonio, who is telegenic and articulate, dispenses a wide variety of medicinal barks, leaves, and roots from the surrounding forest. Some TV crews go no further than Antonio's ideally situated herbal emporium.

As we arrived at Antonio's shop, a Japanese TV crew was finishing up a shot of the numerous medicinal plants there. "This is a very convenient place," Antonio explained to Bernie and me. "You don't have to go hiking off into the bush. There are many good medicines here." Once the TV crew had packed up their gear and departed, Antonio told us about the various plants he used and sold. "I have many collectors who bring in different plants from all over, some even very far away. They know that I only take good quality. The people who come to see me for help and advice get very good remedies. I am carrying on a family tradition here, and I want to provide the best natural medicines possible."

Bernie explained that I was researching sex plants, and Antonio smiled at that. I asked Antonio if there was any single herb that he thought was the very best for sexual enhancement. He pointed straight away to a wooden bin containing sections of dried bark. "There is nothing that compares with catuaba. I have used this plant with many people, for a very long time. The old become sexually young again. I have given catuaba to impotent men, and they can have sex for the first time in years. Even healthy couples find that catuaba puts extra fire in their sex life." Antonio expressed his opinion that "Catuaba is good for men and women, and no harm can come from taking it." I asked Antonio if he used catuaba himself. He nodded. "Sometimes."

Prior to my trip to the Brazilian Amazon with Bernie, I had acquainted myself with catuaba. The bark of the tree has been widely consumed among the natives of the northern Amazon River basin for centuries to increase libido and improve sexual potency. The harvesting and sale of this plant has become big business throughout Brazil.

I asked Antonio if the popularity of catuaba had harmed the supply. "Yes," he said and nodded thoughtfully. "The trees were very abundant around here. But now so many people have cut them down, there's not much left. So now most of the catuaba is coming from Rondonia, farther south." The World Health Organization identifies this as a problem that native cultures face all over the world. When a plant becomes popular, many people harvest that plant to supplement meager incomes. You can't blame them at all for doing so. But often this practice damages wild supplies and endangers natural habitat. I asked if anybody was planting catuaba. "Yes, in Rondonia. That's the only way we're going to prevent them from completely disappearing. More and more people want better sexual health, so there is only going to be increased demand."

Bernie told us both that Rondonia is the original home of his tribe, the Eur-eu-wa-wa. "That's way the heck in the forest, man. Maybe we can still find what we're looking for closer to here. Otherwise we're going to have a very long trip."

I asked Antonio's recommendation for the best way to take catuaba. "You mix a teaspoon of the powdered bark in about three fingers of water. To make this mixture even more potent, you can add a teaspoon of powdered guarana (*Paulinia cupana*). If you take this drink once daily before eating, you will have the sexual vitality of a much younger person." Antonio further explained that some people also made a wine in which the bark of catuaba is soaked for three weeks, and then the strained herbal wine infusion is drunk. "You can drink a glass of that wine every day, and it will make you sexually very strong." Women too? I asked. "Yes, definitely for women too.

Many women come in here for increased sexual energy, not just men. Catuaba helps them."

One of Antonio's sons, who works at his father's business, offered to arrange a meeting with a catuaba dealer named Sivao. We settled on a time in two days and said good-bye, allowing Antonio to turn back to the work of advising people about their health, and providing them with rain forest remedies.

Hot Plant of the Northern Amazon

According to tribal lore, the Tupi Indians in Brazil first discovered the aphrodisiac properties of catuaba. Indigenous peoples have used catuaba for generations. Catuaba is not only a sex-enhancing botanical. Natives in the northern Amazon use catuaba as a central nervous stimulant and general tonic, and it is often employed after illness to restore health and vitality. A decoction of the bark is administered to treat nervousness and poor memory. Without question the most popular uses of catuaba are for treating sexual impotence and boosting diminished desire.

Erythroxylum catuaba is a small, vigorous-growing tree with yellow and orange flowers, which grows in the northern part of Brazil. The catuaba tree grows between 2–4 meters in height and belongs to the same botanical family (*Erythroxylaceae*) as coca, the source of cocaine. Despite this familial bond, catuaba contains none of that stimulant drug. The bark of catuaba contains aromatic oils, resins, and sterols. The compounds believed to most directly affect sexual function are two alkaloids, catuabine A and catuabine B.

Animal studies on catuaba demonstrate antibacterial and antiviral properties. In mice, catuaba extract provided protection against infections of the dangerous bacteria Escherichia coli and Staphlococcus aureus, and also inhibited HIV. Many plant extracts show some inhibitory activity against HIV. This does not mean that they are proven cures for HIV, or effective in any way against AIDS. But it is entirely possible that one or more plant-derived drugs will eventually add to the arsenal of doctor-prescribed anti-HIV agents that help to maintain quality of life among the infected.

No clinical studies have yet addressed the use of catuaba as an aphrodisiac, but the widespread consumption of catuaba bark preparations for sexual purposes by large numbers of natives over many generations is ample testimony to the plant's efficacy. Like so many traditional native remedies, catuaba's use was once exclusive to those tribal populations where the tree grows. Today, catuaba is popular in the European and U.S. markets in capsules and in fluid extracts.

Super Sex Shakes

Bernie and I stayed in a Manaus hotel for two nights so we could peruse the numerous local markets for regional herbal remedies, and to check out the popular use of another Amazonian plant, guarana. Though Brazil is a huge coffee producing nation, guarana is the most popular caffeine-bearing plant in the country. Guarana is the dried seed paste of *Paulinia cupana,* a bushy tree that grows both wild and cultivated in the upper Amazon basin. Guarana seed paste contains 2.5–5 percent caffeine and is a common ingredient in soft drinks, syrups, and guarana sticks. These sticks, which look like brown dynamite, are scraped on a grater, and the resulting powder is added to beverages.

Around Manaus, stores and street carts featured a wide variety of guarana-based sodas. Though the U.S. market favors heavy-tasting colas flavored with the caffeine-bearing cola nut, Brazilians prefer the lighter and more delicate taste of guarana. Some pale sodas we encountered were labeled as guarana "champagnes." Those sodas possessed a clean, pleasing flavor and effervesced with a profusion of tiny bubbles.

Bernie and I came upon dozens of guarana stands. These blender-drink shops feature brilliant yellow awnings, with GUARANA written in huge letters. They serve mixed fruit smoothies blended with guarana powder, and some popular drinks contain additional herbs. The guarana stands offer a variety of drinks in which powdered guarana seed paste is blended with exotic fruits like acai, buriti, cupuacu, mango, and papaya. These sweet, energizing fruit smoothies are highly popular. At busy times, lines of customers at guarana stands are a common sight.

The menu of one guarana stand we saw offered a "Super Sex Drink," which contained a heaping teaspoon of guarana powder, plus a heaping teaspoon of powdered catuaba bark blended with any of the region's tropical fruits. This was one of the most popular of all the drinks, according to a young man behind the counter. I ordered one, and Bernie looked at me. "What are you going to do with that? You got no woman here, you're going to climb the walls later on." I replied that field-work has its intrinsic hazards and signaled the counter help to fire up a blender and make me a drink.

The people who worked at the guarana stands we visited

had many tales to share concerning the Super Sex Drink, which turned out to be on every menu. One especially beautiful woman at a stand told me about a hundred-year-old man who consumed a Super Sex Drink and then went home and chased his centenarian wife around the bedroom. I doubted the story at once, but that didn't prevent me from laughing at the image it conjured. At guarana stands we saw couples buying sex drinks together and smiling at each other suggestively as they drank. Men and women individually consumed the herbal potions on the spot, and took more home in plastic bottles to their partners. Overall, the guarana stands in Manaus did a brisk trade in sex drinks.

That night after consuming the super sex shake, I awoke with an unrelenting erection. The catuaba had worked very well indeed. I noted its strong activity with some chagrin, but was glad to know first hand that the plant worked. Getting back to sleep proved somewhat difficult, and I decided to forego any more super sex shakes as long as I had no partner with whom to share the benefits.

Black River

After a couple of days in Manaus, Bernie and I collected our belongings and headed to the crowded docks behind the Mercado. "It's gonna be very easy to find a boat," Bernie explained. "These guys are eager to take you anywhere, for one hour or for two weeks, it's what they do." We descended long stairs to the waterfront and walked along looking at various crafts, from triple decker riverboats to rowboats. All around us dock workers labored, many with huge palettes on their heads, laden with bananas, fish, cilantro, scallions, and fruits. Most were short and muscular and seemed to carry their unwieldy and heavy loads with relative ease. Vendors walked from boat to boat, hawking soda, bread, beer, fruit, cooked meats and fish. The atmosphere was lively. At one neat blue wooden boat about eighteen feet long, a deeply tanned man with a friendly smile called out to us. "He's asking if we want a ride," Bernie translated. Minutes later, we reached a mutually satisfactory agreement with a man named Pedro Roque, who told us that he had worked the Amazon River and the Rio Negro as a boatman for over twenty years.

Bernie and I asked Pedro to take us up the Rio Negro, where according to Antonio, we were reasonably certain to find catuaba. "I know many good villages up there," Pedro said. "I can take you to some, and maybe you will find what you are looking for. Many people up the river know the plants very well." And so we set off, first on the vast Amazon River out of Manaus, then turning north up the Rio Negro. I marveled at the water, which flowed clean and black, colored from the pigments of plant sediment. As we motored north, black freshwater dolphins leapt beside us, and periodically we saw large, bright pink dolphins, which breached the river's surface and slipped with easy dives below and out of sight. The banks of the river displayed a riot of emerald rain forest plant life, with trees small and large crowding each other for a place in the sun.

For many hours we rode up river. At one point, the sky filled with clouds, and a heavy rainstorm pelted us so hard Pedro had to steer his boat into a huge floating clump of grasses several acres in size and stay put until the storm broke. Following the intense rain we were treated to a spectacular dome rainbow. Along the river banks, large alligators lay half submerged, their eyes above the water line and part of their spikey backs exposed.

"You see those guys," Bernie said, pointing to the alligators. "A lot of the time, they will come up under a canoe, and just knock it over. Many natives die that way. Those alligators are very smart." I filed away the information in my mind for future canoe rides in those waters.

We traveled with Pedro for about six hours, deeper into the rain forest, occasionally passing small villages and children on the river banks. I shot rolls and rolls of photographs. Most of the way, the river stretched a couple of miles across. We traveled a few hundred yards from the eastern bank. Small brilliant blue birds flew inches above floating purple flowers, and entire flocks of bright green parrots arced from one tree to another. Eventually we came to an *igarape',* a small river, and turned into it. From there our passage was five or six hundred feet across. Large numbers of fish leaped from the surface of the water. After another half hour or so, Pedro steered his boat toward a sandy beach where eight wooden huts stood side by side on the rise of a hill. "I know these people," Pedro told us. "This is a good village. Plus, they will cook the chicken I have brought. There are people here who know the plants in the surrounding forest."

Bernie winked at me. "See that, big guy? We get lunch and maybe our catuaba too." The little village seemed a million miles away from anything, and I was happy to get out of the boat and stretch my legs. "First we go see the chief," Bernie told me. "Then, the women will make food for us." We tied Pedro's boat to a tree and headed up a path to look for the village chief, who proved easy to find. Wearing a ragged baseball cap and a faded green T-shirt with a number of rips in it, the chief sat drinking coffee in a shack close to the woods, and near a *fugao,* a large outdoor oven used to prepare manioc, the staple starch food of that region. He invited us to sit and have coffee. That offer set in motion four charming and smiling women who fussed over us, gave us cups and coffee and sugar, and placed some dense homemade manioc flatcakes before us.

Bernie explained who we were, and why we were in the Amazon, while Pedro negotiated the cooking of lunch with one of the women in the shack. The chief, whose name was Jose, told us that we were welcome to stay there overnight, and that just a bit farther up the river he knew of a place where an old man knew all the plants in the region. He was sure we would find our catuaba. Bernie looked at me. "I guess we're just going to have to take the chief up on his offer of hospitality, and eat some lunch and relax." That seemed okay to me, and Pedro was happy for the plan.

Domingo's Catuaba

We passed a lovely evening and night in the small village, sleeping in hammocks strung to the rafters of an old wooden schoolhouse. The next morning, after coffee and more manioc flatbread, we left some money for the village and set off again further up river, to a place the chief had directed us. "There is an old man there, he is a very well-respected shaman. He can take you to find the plants you seek."

After about an hour of travel, we pulled up to another small sand beach and walked up a hill to a shack. There we inquired about the shaman. "Oh, he is gone to Manaus," the woman there told us. "His son was injured, and so the old man went to the hospital." When would he return? we inquired. "Oh, I don't know. Maybe a week." I wasn't particularly disappointed, as plans change all the time on the medicine trail. I assumed that we would encounter another plant expert. Nearby another shack stood where a man was cleaning the counter of what appeared to be a small store. Pedro suggested that we have a beer, and so we walked over.

The man behind the counter, whose name was Domingo, asked us who we were and what we were doing. Once again Bernie told the tale. When he was finished, the man said, "Well, I'm not a shaman, but I know some of the plants around here because I have lived here my whole life. I can take you to see catuaba, no problem." Domingo suggested that we have a beer and relax awhile, and then he would take us into the forest.

Into the Forest

About two hours later, Domingo, Bernie, Pedro, and I set off into the forest to seek catuaba. It was the middle of the day, and the equatorial sun produced sweltering heat. In the mottled light of the forest interior, luminous blue morpho butterflies and brightly colored birds flew in and out of the shadows. Trees held great termite nests and beehives. Lizards scampered up trunks. A large iguana sunned itself passively on the end of a denuded branch overhead as we walked quietly through the jungle.

The smells of the forest were an olfactory riot of butter-scotch, honeysuckle, watermelon, lemon, mildew, moldy bark, meat, and feces. Every few feet we encountered a new aroma. The jungle offered a profusion of floral, carnal, and sometimes indescribable olfactory sensations.

I paid special attention to sharp thorns, which seemed to be everywhere. Trees, bushes, and grasses bore thorns of all sizes.

Some trees had short, fat spikes. Others were covered with long, hard needles the size of eight penny nails. Long grasses bore needle-sharp thorns on their undersides. Tiny, soft-looking thorns on broad-leafed plants delivered irritating pricks to the skin. We were constantly ducking thorny foliage or carefully pushing it out of the way.

As we hiked along in the forest, we brushed against branches and leaves and took on spiders by the dozens. The number and diversity of spiders was fascinating. Tiny spiders no bigger than grains of sand hiked up and down my arms on filamentous legs. Awkward daddy long legs walked on spindly appendages over our shirts and hats. Sturdier blue, brown, orange, and gray spiders leapt onto us, scrambled on our bodies and faces, climbed up our necks, and leapt onto branches that brushed us. Some spiders moved slowly, while others possessed astonishing speed. Furry spiders half the size of my hand climbed all over nearby trees.

All the while we were a walking meal to thousands of gnats and mosquitoes. Vicious-looking wasps flew at us, finding nothing of interest, and moved on. In small patches of light, dozens of metallic blue dragonflies hovered in the air, rapidly beating delicate veined wings. A small preying mantis climbed slowly and awkwardly up the back of Bernie's shirt. I repeatedly glanced down at my feet to see a dozen hungry gnats feeding on my flesh. I mashed them all with a rough swipe of my hand and repeated the process every minute or so.

As Domingo led us through the thick jungle, I watched for any poisonous green snakes that might be hanging from branches. "You know, man," Bernie said, "I got bitten one time by a green snake, right on the side of my neck. They like to go for this area. He was hanging from a tree, and he bit me right here. I got sick, but thank the great spirit I didn't die. I think it was a dry bite." Dry bites, not uncommon, occur when poisonous vipers sink their fangs into a person or animal, but inject no venom.

Domingo kept apologizing for not being a shaman, but he seemed to know almost every plant we passed. "This one here is for very bad headaches," he would say. "You scrape the inner bark and make a dark brown tea and drink it, and the headaches go." We would walk another few feet and Domingo would point again. "If you collect the sap from this vine, it will soothe a very sick stomach." He was quick to add, "But I'm not a shaman. A good shaman would know much more than I do." It was like that for a long way as we threaded through the jungle. We collected numerous plant samples, and I personally marveled at Domingo's impressive fluency in the local flora.

After a short while, Domingo halted before a small tree with bright yellow flowers. "There is your catuaba," he declared. I asked Domingo if there was much catuaba left in that region. "Yes, still a pretty good amount," he said. "Not as many people collect catauaba here as they do closer to Manaus, so we still have a lot in the woods. I asked Domingo if he ever used catuaba. "Sure," he told me. "It makes your cock hard like wood. Everybody uses catuaba. The women like it too. They like how lusty it makes them feel. It is good if you have somebody to make love with. Otherwise, it is too strong." I was happy to see catuaba growing in its natural habitat but had no need to take any from the forest, as Antonio had already provided us with a couple of kilos' worth of dried bark. We continued our walk through the forest and saw several other catuaba trees as we made our way.

Theresa's Advice

Four days later, Bernie and I were down the Amazon River with his adopted family, a charming and friendly group of Ipixuna Indians. In the company of several members of his family, we set off to see a renowned shaman named Theresa, who lived off the river in the small and crumbling town of Iranduba. We walked for a mile or more through high shiny grass with blades as sharp as knives. The sun baked us as we went. Lizards scampered across our path, and occasionally a group of birds erupted from the grass and flew off. After about an hour of walking, we came to a small and tidy yellow house. One of the Ipixuna women, Jeriza, knew shaman Theresa, so she led the way into the old woman's home and introduced us all. Theresa invited us to sit with her and began to tell us of her work healing people who came to her from far and wide. "Sometimes they hear about me very far away, but they come, because I have a good reputation. I know the plants in the forest well, and most of the time I can help people to be well again."

I asked Theresa about catuaba, and whether she used it in her practice. "Oh, yes, it is the most effective plant for sex. Many men and women lose their desire, and so I give them catuaba. It makes them want to be sexual again. Women lose desire later in life, and catuaba brings it back like when they were young. Also men come because they can no longer achieve an erection. Usually after using catuaba for just a little while, they feel young again and they are able to have sex."

What is the best way to prepare catuaba? I inquired. "Well, you take a glass of water, and you put a small handfull of bark into it. You let that water sit overnight, and in the morning you drink the water. That is one good way. The other way is to put the bark in wine, and drink that wine every day, not too much, just one cup or so. Even if you are very low in desire, or are having problems, the catuaba will restore you."

Theresa went on to say that other plants in the Amazon were also good for enhancing sex. One, muirapuama (*Ptychopetalum olacoides*), was actually the subject of an erectile function study in men. Also a tree, the muirapuama significantly improved sexual function in the study. Guarana, the caffeine-bearing Amazonian berry, was also widely used for sexual enhancement. "But none of them are as good as catuaba. Catuaba is the top plant for sex. It makes you sexually young again."

Using Catuaba

Bernie and I traveled for about three weeks, visiting a number of herbal experts. All agreed that catuaba was the most effective Amazonian plant for boosting sexual desire and function. One of the challenges of translating traditional herbal remedies into reliably effective modern products concerns dosage. No specific dosage such as "500 milligrams per day" or any other accurate measure has been established. Leslie Taylor of the Amazonian medicinal herb company Raintree, says that "recommended usage is reported to be 1–3 cups of an infusion daily, or 2–3 ml of a standard alcohol tincture twice daily." I have seen products containing 500 milligrams of powdered catuaba bark per dose, and even more. You will find products on the market which are in capsules, tablets, and fluid extracts. The basic rules apply: use products from reputable companies, and assiduously avoid those from companies without a good reputation or those making questionable claims. You can find information about supplement companies in *Consumer Reports,* or you can also ask personnel in natural food stores about quality brands.

Experts in Amazonian herbs agree that catuaba demonstrates no health hazards, so some experimentation is in order to determine the dose that works for you. When you hit that dose, you will know that catuaba, the hot plant of the Amazon, is working for you.

THE PERFUMED GARDEN

Zallouh, Ferulis Harmonis

YOU COULD SAY THAT BY SEXUAL STANDARDS, KING SOLOMON had it made. He enjoyed intimate relations with seven hundred wives, surely a staggering number by any standard, and all of them gorgeous and exotic. The wives of King Solomon's harem lived an opulent existence, in a splendid Arabian oasis of tall palms and golden sands and clear springs. These beautiful women dallied and sported in cavernous white marble halls. Princesses and sultans' daughters cooled themselves with sweet, delicate sherbets in the heat of the desert sun and passed the cold moonlit nights of winter together.

The women feasted on platters of fresh figs and sticky, black dates the size of a large man's thumb. They nibbled on delicate tarts and fritters, Omani peaches, Sultani oranges, Palmyra pomegranates, and Tihama raisins. They licked the juices of fresh roast mutton off their delicate manicured fingers and sipped lightly from golden goblets of rare strained wines. They ate salty jumbo olives packed in brine and oil, sugared squash blossoms, hard Damascus cheese, and desserts of melon preserves and candied ginger and lady's fingers piled high on earthen platters.

The inner harem was filled with fresh flowers far from Solomon's vast kingdom, and the air was redolent with the narcotic fragrance of narcissus and the glorious perfumes of Aleppine jasmine, orchids, freesias, Damascene nenuphars, scented myrtle berries, delicate tea roses, and violets. Immense bouquets crowned sculpted glass pedestals and pillars of rose marble. Garlands and wreaths of blossoms on threads of colored silks adorned pillows and doors and tables.

Solomon's wives smelled like no other women in the world, scented with the costliest fragrances of the perfumer's art. They wore real musk, ambergris, and civet, ylang ylang, coriander and cardamom oils, sandalwood, Persian amber, and Constantinople rose. Their fragrant effusion wafted and circulated on slow, lazy breezes as they walked the sunny courtyards and cool, shaded hallways of the inner palace.

The wives were guarded by fierce broad-shouldered blackamoors wearing gigantic turbans and armed with razor-sharp scimitars, who were trained to cleave a man in half with one deft stroke. As much as the wives lay safe and protected from intruders, they were also cloistered in splendor, cut off from the world, living in servitude to the king.

And for Solomon's pleasure, the women of the harem prepared for the king infused goblets of Shirsh Zallouh, a hairy-rooted plant from the heights of Mount Haramoun. This drink, it is said, imbued the king with extraordinary virility, enabling him to enter into sexual congress with several wives in a night.

If we believe legend, King Solomon was better able to enjoy the amorous pleasures of his wives due to the invigorating effects of a legendary hot plant, Shirsh Zallouh. But where did this plant originate, and how was its use discovered? In this instance, we can thank goats. In the Middle East, the discovery of a number of plants, including coffee, is attributed to goats. We can credit their omnivorous appetite with the discovery of Shirsh Zallouh. No other agent occupies such a high place in that region for boosting sexual capacity.

According to legend, a goatherd tending his flock high up on the rocky slopes of Mount Haramoun noticed that when his animals nibbled on the green tops of a particular mountain plant, they became sexually rambunctious, copulating with great vigor and frequency. The goatherd marveled at the sexual antics of the animals and sought the advice of a learned scholar who knew the uses of many plants. Not long after, the scholar experimented with the green plant, discovering that the root especially produced a powerful feeling of sexual excitement. Soon all the people in the goatherd's community learned that when they ate from the same plant, they too became sexually invigorated. Naturally, word spread about the plant's remarkable effects. Today that particular green-topped plant from atop Mount Haramoun is known as *Ferulis harmonis,* or zallouh.

The tale of zallouh's discovery by goats points to the fact that, in many cases, animal behavior has led to the discovery of beneficial, health-imbuing plants. This is part of the human plant discovery process that has spanned at least 60,000 years. Zallouh has been highly revered since ancient times. One tale has it that around 1000 B.C., King Solomon and Makeda, the Queen of Sheba, built a temple near the base of Mount Haramoun to honor zallouh. Though this oft-repeated legend flies in the face of historical record, it points to the exceptionally high status of this sex-enhancing plant.

What is this plant?

Zallouh (*Ferulis harmonis*) is a small shrub with thin leaves and tiny white or yellow flowers. Zallouh is a member of the parsley family. Also commonly known as "Shirsh Zallouh" the plant grows between 6,000 and 10,000 feet around massive Mount Haramoun, which straddles the borders of Syria, Lebanon, and Israel. In that region, the plant is extravagantly profuse. At present, many thousands of tons of zallouh grow on Mount Haramoun. Conditions do not make harvesting the plant entirely safe. Due to ongoing ethnic and religious conflicts in the Middle East, the Israeli side of Mount Haramoun is not a safe or secure source of zallouh. On the Lebanese side, indiscriminate harvesting of the wild plant has reduced its occurence. As a result, the Lebanese government has made efforts to limit zallouh harvesting. In Syria, a nation under military rule, zallouh trade is overseen by the Syrian Army, and the harvesting of zallouh is conducted in a controlled, sustainable fashion. The root is typically harvested from August to October.

Though the legend of zallouh's discovery concerns goats eating the green tops of the plant, it is the hairy, somewhat bitter root of the plant that has been employed as a sex enhancer since antiquity. Zallouh has a long tradition of use by men with erectile problems, and for both men and women with low libido. The root has also enjoyed even broader use for sexual enhancement among healthy men and women, to increase sexual frequency, and to increase pleasure. Zallouh makes users want to spend more time making love and adds a thrilling dimension to sex, greatly enhancing sensation. Zallouh has a well-deserved reputation as an aphrodisiac. Not just a remedy for sexual dysfunction, zallouh is an agent for boosting sexual urges in healthy individuals and adding extra pleasure to amorous activity. Hneiny, a Lebanese pharmaceutical company, has described the use of zallouh by men and women in this way: "They mostly come in complete secrecy to cure their frigidity, impotence or those of their sons who cannot satisfy their brides sexually. . . . They come back stunned by the miracles achieved which they would never have dared to dream of!"

Almost every week we are made aware through exuberant media of yet another herb that is supposed to supercharge sexual function. Zallouh has been boldly proclaimed an "herbal Viagra," or a "sexual fountain of youth." It has been the subject of a flattering report on CNN, and in numerous newspaper articles. Zallouh lives up to the description. I was first made aware of zallouh by Travis Hammond of Nutranex, a maker of zallouh products distributed in the United States. Travis asked if I would be interested in conducting field research on this plant. After reviewing the literature he provided, the decision was easy. I booked passage to Beirut, Lebanon, to find out for myself what I could about this hot plant.

The Zallouh King

Beirut, Lebanon, offers a strange and unsettling juxtaposition of architectural styles. On the one hand, hundreds of buildings in the city are riddled with bullet holes or partly bombed to pieces, a result of the war of 1975–1990, which devastated the city. As developers have erected splendid new hotels, apartment buildings, office towers, and residences, the city is undergoing a transformation, a reincarnation. There is a sense of new energy, of the irrepressible nature of life and hope, which can spring anew even from the crumbled ruins of a broken place.

Beirut is a bustling metropolis, where madcap taxi drivers fly about and trucks of all sizes race through the streets as if they are storming the city, the former "Paris of the Middle East."

My first mission was a search for the king of zallouh, Dr. Pierre Malychef. In the Jal Eldib area of Beirut, Dr. Pierre Malychef operates a pharmacy near Aboujaoude Hospital. Finding an address in Beirut isn't easy; many streets lack signs, and numbers on buildings are few and far between. My taxi driver stopped several times to ask directions, and there was a lot of conversation, gesticulating, and pointing before we eventually pulled up to the right spot. The store stood as a shrine to Lebanon's most famous plant, zallouh. Signs and displays proudly proclaimed the numerous invigorating health benefits of the plant, and various newspaper and magazine articles on zallouh from around the world festooned the pharmacy walls. Dr. Malychef can take credit for almost all of zallouh's fame, which has resulted from his own tireless promotion of what he considers to be an elixir of life and vitality. A pharmacist for more than fifty years, Malychef is a specialist in phytotherapy, pharmacology, and toxicology. More than any other person in the Middle East, he has championed the health benefits of zallouh.

Dr. Malychef is used to visitors and reporters. When I told him that I had traveled from the United States to see him, he nodded with the practiced appreciation of a man who had heard it many times before. "Yes," Malychef told me. "Many people come to speak with me, always about zallouh." He grinned broadly. As his fame has spread, TV crews from CNN and other news outfits from around the world have shown up at his door. "Shirsh Zallouh is much more than a sex plant," Malychef declared right at the start. "It is very good for that purpose, and I have given it to many, many people who have been satisfied. But it also contains antioxidants, and it helps to retard the aging process. If you will take zallouh every day, it will help to keep you strong and youthful." Malychef was in fact making claims for zallouh similar to those for other hot plants such as *Rhodiola rosea* and ashwagandha, which are adaptogens. These plants not only enhance sexual function, but provide a wide range of additional restorative and invigorating benefits.

At seventy-seven years old, Pierre Malychef attributed much of his evident vitality and fitness to zallouh. In a small lab in the pharmacy, Malychef painstakingly manufactures his own extracts of zallouh root in small but highly potent batches. His son Alexi travels to remote villages on the Lebanese side of Mount Haramoun, where he collects zallouh for extraction in Beirut. In the lab at the back of his pharmacy, Pierre Malychef produces the elixirs that have made his shop the most celebrated pharmacy in Beirut.

To show me how he prepared zallouh, Malychef cut up a large root with a long knife and put the herb into a round glass flask partly filled with alcohol and water, to transform it into the local wonder drug. "I am making an extract of this root by a very special and scientific method, using hot extraction and distillation," Malychef explained. Lighting a small gas flame under the flask, Malychef studied the contents as the mixture started to bubble. "This is an effective extract, with no side effects and only one slight problem. The taste is a little rough, quite bitter, really. It's good to put it in milk or fruit juice and it should be acceptable." I immediately asked to taste a sample of the straight extract.

"You sure?" asked Malychef. After I insisted, the silver-haired pharmacist poured a small amount of amber extract from a bottle into a cup and handed it to me. I downed the liquid, pausing to give a good taste. It wasn't bad. Along the medicine trail I have tasted far, far worse. As a researcher I try sometimes repugnant potions, from infusions of snakes to potions made with ground insects and pressed reptiles. Zallouh extract tasted rather pleasant to me by comparison.

In Malychef's crowded pharmacy, several zallouh preparations were displayed, including a scalp rub which he insisted would renew hair growth. I didn't want to point out that his own hair, while a lovely silver, was sparse. The most popular of all Malychef's zallouh products is the concentrated liquid extract for sexual enhancement. "We go through a lot of this," Malychef boasted. "Once somebody tries zallouh extract for sexual vigor, they come back for more, because it is very, very effective. Men and women both use the extract, and they keep coming back. This is the thing about plants. They really do possess powerful healing properties. People discover for themselves just how effective an herb can be, and then they understand. Plants are so much more in harmony with our bodies than any drugs can ever be."

I asked him about the use of zallouh for impotence and erectile problems. "Yes, many people come here because they are having sexual problems. It is probably the very number-one reason that people come in here. I see a lot of that. After these people use zallouh for a while, they are usually better. Many people tell me that any sexual difficulties they had were successfully eliminated with zallouh. It is unquestionably a sexual wonder. I have not seen any other plant which revitalizes people the way that zallouh does."

Human Clinical Studies

Zallouh has also undergone scientific clinical study. In Beirut, the Lebanese Urological Society has sponsored clinical trials that have brought this traditional root of antiquity into the medical present. The Lebanese government is keenly supportive of zallouh, and this has led to a series of human studies, conducted on a large scale. To date more than 7,000 men have participated in this research.

In the studies conducted on zallouh, we see firsthand a bias that is prevalent in the Middle East. Men and women in the Middle East are as sexually active and sexually interested as any people, but there is a significant taboo against any explicit acknowledgment of female sexuality in the majority of nations in that region. The human clinical studies on zallouh root have been conducted only on men. No study has ever focused on women's sexual needs or function. So we can count solely on the historical and current verbal reports by women about libido enhancement and sexual pleasure to say that zallouh is suitable for both sexes.

Men selected as candidates for trials have uniformly experienced some measure of erectile dysfunction. Either the men have been unable to achieve an erection hard enough to engage in intercourse, or maintain an erection. In one six-month study of 315 men with a mean age of fifty-five, among the 159 who took either 500 or 1,000 milligrams of freeze-dried zallouh root, 80 percent experienced improvement. On a scale of 1 to 5, the men went from an average score of 1.26 (virtually no erection) to an average of 3.11 (a firm erection). To complete the data collection on the study, the researchers conducted a study to evaluate the partners' perceptions of the efficacy of zallouh in patients with erectile dysfunction treated at Malaab Medical Center in Beirut. They presented results from twelve weeks of observation and feedback from spouses or female partners who were asked to record number of successful attempts at sexual intercourse and fill out a two-part questionnaire asking, "How often did he get an erection?" and "How often did he maintain an erection?" Responses were graded on a scale of 1 to 5 ranging from never to always with zero representing no sexual activity.

The responses of the female partners of the males treated with Zallouh correlated closely with results reported by the treated subjects. There was a significant increase in the number of partners reporting improved erections and increased successful attempts at sexual intercourse in the treated group (80 percent) compared to the placebo group (10 percent).

In the largest zallouh study of all, 4,274 patients ages eighteen to eighty-seven participated. Of these, 2,722 took zallouh root, between 2–8 grams daily in the form of tea. At the end of the year, 2,199 patients on zallouh had completed the study, with an efficacy rate nearing 86 percent for improved erectile function. These results are spectacular and show promise for large doses of zallouh taken over an extended period. Not all the studies were as impressive, depending on the dosage of zallouh given and the duration of the study. The lowest efficacy rates in clinical trials hovered around 60 percent, which is still remarkably good, compared with placebo groups at about 10 percent.

How Does It Work?

What is found in zallouh root that so markedly improves erectile function? Proponents of the root point to its content of ferulic acid and feruloside, both of which they claim dilate blood vessels and stimulate circulation. Currently there is no strong scientific data to support this activity by these compounds. We may not know yet what makes zallouh work, but there is no question that the root works very well.

What we do know is that when zallouh is taken, an erection occurs more easily, and the erection is firmer than without zallouh. The root may cause side effects. Those with hypertension, heart disease, or diabetic neuropathy should not take zallouh root without the approval of a physician. Some individuals who take zallouh experience flushing and headaches. This would suggest that something in zallouh increases circulation in fine vessels, thus enhancing erectile function. The same effect should apply to clitoral circulation as well, supporting the use of zallouh root among women. For the most part, zallouh root and its various preparations appear safe and effective for a majority of users.

Zallouh root is not currently standardized to a specific potency of any one compound. But a daily dose of anywhere from 500 milligrams to 1,500 milligrams of the freeze-dried root concentrate will put you right in the zone of maximum efficacy. Even though all studies on zallouh have been conducted with men, female use reputedly goes a long way back in time. According to Dr. Pierre Malychef, women who use zallouh find the plant every bit as sexually stimulating as do men.

In the Souqs

Strolling past the massive stone Roman-era Citadel in Old Damascus, Syria, I turned into Souq al-Hamidiyeh, a long and cobbled marketplace covered by a corrugated iron roof.

Shopkeepers invited me into their stores to consider every kind of dry good, from trousers to carpets, fine fabrics, ornately carved and inlaid tables, and Roman coins. Sparkling brass pots finely engraved with Arabesque designs filled traditional craft shop windows. Exquisite pieces of art depicting brave warriors and lovely women adorned the walls of numerous small galleries. Other stores displayed batteries and plastic ware, stacks of underwear and socks, and knockoffs of popular western athletic footware.

From Souq al-Hamidiyeh, I headed to the massive and ornate Umayyad Mosque, where a steady flow of people were entering that splendid and palatial marble site of worship. Once inside, I discovered that it was acceptable to photograph inside the grand mosque. I shot several photographs of the splendid golden mosaics that covered the courtyard walls.

After taking in the sights and echoing sounds of the mosque, and pigeons flying about and children calling out to one another, I kept on my way, heading first into the Al Bzouriya souq, into a labyrinth of old markets, alleys that led into other alleys and led into still others, deep in the older parts of that oldest city. In those souqs I passed great sacks of coffee beans, tables piled high with platters of olives of every size, green and black, oil cured and brined, some with pimiento, some with herbs, many glistening with fresh oil. Other stalls sold cheeses in wedges and wheels, stacked high atop one another. Some cheeses sat flecked with herbs, others lay partly submerged in golden olive oil. Still others hung in nets from the ceiling. Other stalls displayed colorful herbs of various kinds, for cooking and scenting and for use as folk medicines. Lavender and valerian sat beside cumin and fenugreek, peppermint and chamomile.

The large open bins of herbs were colorful to look at and fragrant to smell.

I stopped at one especially well-stocked herbal stall and discovered that the vendor possessed a rudimentary command of English. I described to the fellow that I was in search of Shirsh Zallouh. The bearded merchant smiled broadly and produced a bucket from beside the counter, filled with large, hairy, dried zallouh roots. I selected two roots to buy, and the merchant summoned a boy from a tea stall over to his herbal stand. A quick verbal exchange followed, and the boy headed back to his stall with a few pieces of zallouh root, which he placed in a pot of hot water. The herb vendor invited me to sit, and in a few minutes I was treated to a cup of zallouh root tea with honey. The brew was delicious. The vendor, who had been speaking to me in some English but mostly in slow and sincere Arabic, tightened his fist with his forearm up, the universal sign of an erection. We both laughed, and I sat sipping zallouh tea in one of the oldest marketplaces on earth.

The Syrian Connection

On the outskirts of Damascus, Syria, the government's Productive Projects Administration (PPA) manufactures a number of herbal products into tea bags and capsules. While PPA imports many herbs such as ginseng, echinacea, and valerian, they are especially proud of their major domestic herb, zallouh. PPA is run by the Syrian military, so when I arrived there it was like arriving at a military base. Hundreds of young soldiers in clean army uniforms stood eager and proud to show off their work with beneficial herbs.

My hosts at PPA included Lieutenant Elias Faraoun, the head of export, and Colonel Nabil Khlaf, who runs the entire facility. "In antiquity, zallouh was used as a tonic by many people," explained Colonel Nabil. "Today we have manufactured zallouh in a way which preserves its unique composition, so it can be used by people everywhere."

Elias described how the Syrian zallouh crop is sustainably harvested. "We harvest zallouh roots on Mount Haramoun, which we will show you. We have divided the area up into five sectors. Each year, we pick zallouh root from only one sector. And we only pick the tops of the roots. Then we leave that sector alone for four years. This gives the zallouh ample time to fully regenerate. In this way, the zallouh crop is sustained. We are sensitive to the importance of protecting this plant and its habitat."

In the crisp and precise manner of his rank, Colonel Nabil carefully explained that zallouh, once harvested, is rushed to a freezer at PPA, where it is stored at −40° C (−35° F). When the root is ready for further processing, it is shipped frozen to a freeze-drying facility. The resulting concentrated zallouh root retains all of its natural chemical constituents and contains no additives or preservatives of any kind. Colonel Nabil explained the goal of PPA with zallouh. "We want to make sure that the product we provide is as active as the plant when it is on the mountain. We have definitely achieved that."

The PPA facility is ISO 9000 certified, which means that it conforms to exceptionally high international standards of cleanliness, record-keeping, and good manufacturing practices. As I toured the very large plant with Elias and Colonel Nabil, I was impressed by the strict cleanliness, orderliness, and efficiency of the operation. Young soldiers worked at various sparkling stainless-steel machines, including a production line for filling tea bags with zallouh, boxing and labeling the final product.

Rouas Sheik Hassan, chief chemist at PPA, was the only woman at the facility. Surrounded by advanced analytic equipment, she described quality-control procedures for zallouh. "We test every batch of zallouh, before freezing, after freezing, and after freeze-drying. We make sure that the root is free of heavy metals and bacterial contamination. And we also make sure that the root contains all of its important constituents and that nothing is lost in processing. We have found that of all methods, freeze-drying results in the most potent zallouh product."

After a full tour of PPA, I stepped outside for a long series of photographs. The young soldiers, many just teenagers, were all eager to be photographed together. Like young men everywhere, they hammed for the camera. And they said they wanted to be remembered. "You come back sometime?" asks one young soldier. I tell him that I would enjoy that very much. When I left, a line of smiles and waves trailed behind me.

To the Mountain

Every field research trip comes down to the plant at hand. In a black Range Rover, Elias Faraoun set a course for Mount Haramoun. From many spots in Syria you can see the snow-capped peak of the giant mountain, an imposing presence on the horizon. From Damascus we headed south, toward the northern side of the mountain. Elias navigated increasingly steep, difficult roads as we left the desert and headed into the hills. The landscape was sandy, arid, and stark. Along the way we passed many cherry orchards and olive groves. Birds sang cheerfully, and the roadside was abloom with brilliant orange poppies.

Past the hill town of Bloudan, we climbed ever more steeply, until we arrived at an altitude where the houses were fewer and the hillsides were more rugged. As we hit 2,200 meters (7,217 feet), the hillsides were dotted with thousands of green plants. They could be seen everywhere, in all directions, for as far as the eye could see. "That is zallouh," explained Elias. "Now you see why we are not worried about supply." I had seen the same phenomenon before. Certain plants grow only at particular altitudes, and often not even a few meters below. Plants thrive in those conditions that are optimal for their growth.

Leaving the Range Rover, we climbed up the steep mountainside. I was happy to be surrounded on all sides by the fabled plant. The green tops looked like a cross between parsley and fennel. Elias explained the zallouh harvest to me. "From August to a little past December, the soldiers come up here to harvest zallouh. By that time, the tops, which flower in June and July, are dried out and dying. The active ingredients in the tops go back down into the roots. We harvest about twenty tons or so every year, and we have the capacity to take much more without endangering the zallouh if it becomes more popular."

We spent much of the afternoon wandering through the zallouh. I shot plenty of photographs, and Elias mused about how zallouh has become increasingly well known. "The plant has this special power," he declared earnestly. "From a long time ago it was used by many people. And now, maybe the whole world will know about zallouh." I told Elias that in the age of communication, where knowledge spreads rapidly around the world, he was probably correct.

Using Zallouh

Start with 200–400 milligrams of the freeze-dried extract of zallouh root daily. You may find that is sufficient. If you need more, increase your daily intake in increments of 100 milligrams until you experience the effects you seek.

HIGH PLAINS APHRODISIAC

Maca

MACA IS ONE OF MY FAVORITE HOT PLANTS. MACA DOES NOT originate from a tradition of erotica, and is not mentioned in any exotic love texts. Maca is a vegetable that grows in a some-what nasty place. This humble turnip-shaped member of the mustard family originates from the inhospitable Central Highlands of Peru, a windblown, oxygen-deprived, high-altitude land with poor soil and hail on the best days of summer. This legendary plant from the Inca is, in my opinion, one of the greatest of the hot plants. Maca increases strength, energy, stamina, libido, and sexual function, all at once. It has over 2,000 years of safe use, is nontoxic, and is a staple food. It even tastes good. You can make blender drinks, cookies, and pan-cakes with maca. Maca is an equal opportunity sexual booster, igniting the desire and prowess of men and women alike.

According to Peruvian legend, during the height of their em-pire, Incan warriors would consume maca before entering into battle. The maca imbued them with fierce strength and made the Inca daunting adversaries against other fighters. After conquering any city, the Incan soldiers were prohibited from eating maca, to protect the conquered women from their powerful sexual impulses. From as far back as five hundred years ago, maca's reputation for enhancing strength and libido was already well established in Peru. Maca is a food for epic sex. Among the hot plants, maca is as hot as they get.

In January 1999, *The Miami Herald* ran an article in which they described maca as "Peru's Natural Viagra." Three months before that story broke and began a market frenzy for maca, I was in Peru on behalf of PureWorld Botanicals, the largest herbal extraction company in the United States. "I think you should go there and check out maca for us," company president Natalie Koether said to me one day. By that afternoon, I had tickets. We had known for two years that maca was percolating up from virtual obscurity into greater awareness in the herbal world. It was time to investigate the plant in its home country. Eventually, PureWorld would become the leading extractor and marketer of maca in the world, and maca would become a mainstay in the energy, stamina, and sexual-enhancement categories.

The Maca Man

The way Sergio Cam tells it, his involvement with maca was destined. For several years, Sergio stayed in the United States for six months at a time and worked as a contractor building houses north of San Francisco. He did well in the construction business. But Sergio's fortunes changed after a visit home in Peru. "I was at Nazca one time, and a shaman gave me some maca. He told me that the maca would change things for me and it did." Leaving his lucrative contracting work behind, Sergio took up the maca trade as his calling. "I feel like I am on exactly the right path now," he told me. Sergio Cam became one of Peru's most important and successful maca traders, working full-time with maca growers in the Peruvian highlands. I had flown into Lima, Peru where Sergio picked me up. He had a classic native face, shoulder-length black hair, and an open, friendly smile. I could not have found a more ideal ally. We had a lot of territory to cover viewing the maca scene.

First Maca

About seven hours out of Lima by difficult country roads, Sergio, his wife and two daughters, a shaman named Enriqué and I bathed in hot mineral springs in the mountains. The hot springs were in a splendid and scenic natural place, and the bath soothed me to my bones. After soaking in heavenly hot mineral water, I ambled over to a small bar at the springs that offered herbal teas and blender drinks. A woman was making maca blender drinks combining cooked maca, honey, vanilla extract, and the Peruvian grain quinoa. It seemed an ideal opportunity to try maca for the first time. The delicious drink had a mildly sweet, nutty flavor, and a viscous consistency. I swallowed the first tall glassful and promptly ordered another. The maca drink definitely gave me a vigorous lift, and I felt that I could hike all day.

Maca blender drinks are among the most common ways that maca is consumed in Peru. You can walk into any town, large or small, and find at least one place selling maca blender drinks. I would discover later that many other foods are also made from maca. At stores and stands throughout the country you can find maca cookies, instant maca flan mixes, maca syrups, and maca bottled drinks. Many Peruvian urban dwellers consume maca as a supplement in capsules, and apothecaries in Lima carry a wide array of brands. Most Peruvians who benefit from the plant consume it as a food, sometimes as a breakfast porridge called *mazzamora*. When I had finished my maca drink, I asked the woman behind the bar why most people consumed maca. She blushed a little. "It gives you energy and is also very good for sex, you know."

Maca, the Plant

The South American country of Peru is home to extraordinarily diverse terrain, including stark desert coastline, vast Amazon rain forest, majestic snow-capped Andean peaks, and Titicaca, the world's highest navigable lake. The country is one of the most botanically rich nations in the world, and the Peruvian countryside yields a high volume of agricultural crops. Driving from the coast up into the mountains, you can see asparagus, marigold fields, jasmine plantations, and fruit orchards.

Medicinal plants are also cultivated in Peru, serving the domestic and international markets. Peruvian use of traditional medicinal plants dates back at least two thousand years. In the jungles and Amazon River basin within Peru, shamans and native plant healers employ a large pharmacopoeia of botanicals for medicinal and nutritional purposes. Not all Peru's medicinal plants come from the tropical Amazon. In the windblown, high-altitude Central Highlands, a plant passed down from the Inca is one of the country's most popular of all beneficial botanicals. That plant is maca, the sex and vitality secret of the Inca.

Maca, *Lepidium meyenii,* is the only cruciferous plant native to Peru. Cruciferous plants include rapeseed (the source of canola oil), radish, cauliflower, cabbage, Brussels sprouts, Chinese cabbage, mustard, garden rocket, and watercress. Maca is an annual plant with a rosette of frilly leaves lying close to the ground. The plant produces a turniplike hypocotyl, or tuber, which matures within approximately seven months after seeds are planted. The tubers may be red, green, black, pink, purplish, yellow, or cream colored. Locals in the Peruvian highlands claim that yellow roots are preferable, because they are sweeter. Yellow maca accounts for just over 36 percent of harvest on average. The root of maca is dried and stored before use and will keep for seven years.

Details about the origins of maca are sketchy, but the plant is believed to have been cultivated in the San Blas area of the Junin Plateau of Peru's Central Highlands as far back as 2,000 years ago. When the Spanish arrived in Peru in 1526, they began a campaign of cultural devastation, which ultimately resulted in the demise of the Incan empire. The Inca were sophisticated architects, builders, and cultivators of the land. They were expert artists and metal workers. They had established a highly developed society and worshipped the sun, and their prodigious works, including the splendid structures at Machu Picchu, remain among the wonders of the world to this day. Among the many treasures held by the Inca and garnered by the Spanish was maca. The dried root was so highly regarded by the Inca, it was used as currency.

Maca grows in a limited geographic area at elevations between 3,500 and 4,575 meters (10,000 and 15,000 feet). The primary area of maca cultivation is the Junin Plateau, where approximately four hundred hectares (one thousand acres) of maca were grown in the year of 2000, mostly in small family plots. Agricultural experts predict that the acreage dedicated to maca cultivation will steadily increase to meet vigorous market demand. Former Agriculture Minister Rodolfo Munante says about maca, "This is the perfect crop, because we don't even have to promote it. Private industry has moved right in and is doing the job for us. I expect that we'll reach the maximum number of hectares possible, fifty thousand by early in the next century."

The Junin Plateau is a harsh area for any type of plant cultivation. Temperatures often plunge below zero, large hailstones and slushy snow commonly fall in the summer, the oxygen-thin air induces altitude sickness, the rocky soil supports very little plant life, the wind chaps and bites the skin, and the glaring sun can burn you red in minutes. Maca is one of only two food crops to grow in this altitude range; the other crop is potatoes. The plant is unusually frost-resistant and thrives in bad conditions. The average minimum temperature in the highland area where maca grows is $-1.5°$ C ($28°$ F), and the average maximum temparature is $12°$ C ($62°$ F). Temperatures plunge to $-10°$ C ($14°$ F), and frost is frequent.

Many Peruvians consider maca a panacea, claiming that maca stimulates metabolism, regulates hormonal secretion, and combats anemia. They also say that maca helps to improve memory and fight depression. Maca is promoted as an aphrodisiac, stamina-builder, and fertility-enhancer. Enthusiasts of the plant tout maca as a laxative, which may be attributable to its fiber content, and as a cure for rheumatism and respiratory disorders. Drugstores sell maca in capsules for stamina and improved sexual function. Ongoing science will eventually provide a better understanding of these effects. Perhaps the antidepressive effects of maca are due to its magnificent libido-boosting and pleasure-enhancing effects. It's hard to feel down when you are having exhilarating sex.

Though claims have been made for maca, only a few have been corroborated in a lab or clinical setting. In animal experiments, rodents fed maca showed increased energy and stamina, and exhibited a significant increase in sexual activity as compared with those that had not been fed maca. Maca increased sperm production radically in rodents as well. Though no formal studies have been conducted on maca's use for balancing hormone levels in menopausal women, a number of Peruvian physicians claim success with maca for this purpose.

The Expert Speaks

Outside of the chaos that characterizes Lima, the Universidad Nacional Agraria occupies a scenic spot, with trees and flowers and peaceful grounds. Sergio and I traveled there to meet one of the top experts on maca in the world, Professor Rolando Aliaga Cardenas of the Horticulture Department.

In a neat office, we were greeted by Professor Cardenas. On the office walls were area maps of high-altitude Peruvian locations marked with red and yellow, denoting maca cultivation. I asked Professor Cardenas about maca and why it is so popular in Peru. "Well, this plant is a very nutritious food. You know, the International Plant Genetic Resources Institute is very keen to promote maca, because it is a valuable food source in the highlands. Nothing much grows there but potatoes and grasses, but maca does well. And people can use it for many purposes. Mostly they grind it into a flour, and then they cook and bake with that. So maca is highly versatile. You see, probably back in the sixteenth and seventeenth centuries, maca was even much more widely cultivated. And then maca farming diminished. But now of course it is coming back." Why was that? I asked. Cardenas smiled. "This plant has a very significant sexual effect. There is no denying that this is so. Anyone can feel it. And now especially with all the talk about Viagra, maca is becoming even more popular for sexual purposes. Maca is not just a highland peasant food. Now it is very much sought after. And the supply must increase."

I asked Cardenas what he imagined for the future of maca. "There are really two aspects of this. One is that much more maca must be cultivated to meet growing demand. The Junin Plateau is very good for this, and I think that over the next few years the acreage there dedicated to maca will increase a great deal. But we are also looking at the area around Lake Titicaca, as it is at a high altitude and similar in its overall conditions. I think it will be possible to grow many thousands of acres of maca over time. But right now, we are limited in this effort by the amount of seed available. We cannot just build the acreage up dramatically, because there is simply not enough seed to plant. So we must increase cultivation a bit at a time and slowly build up the total volume."

What was the second aspect of maca's future? "You will see some very significant companies, extraction companies, and pharmaceutical companies, taking a very good look at maca. I can tell you that already now some companies are working with the plant, identifying various phytochemicals which may be of great health value. They are figuring out ways to make more effective and concentrated maca products. So I think that scientific development will move maca along to a position of higher demand as well."

Maca and the Spanish

Maca may have been an Incan treasure, but nobody outside of that empire knew about it until Spanish conquistadores ventured into the high altitude of Peru's Central Highlands. There the Spanish became concerned for the health and fertility of their livestock, especially their horses. In the highlands there were no grasslands for grazing, and the thin air and hostile climate produced a precipitous drop in animal fertility. The Inca recommended that the Spanish feed their horses the root-like maca, which grew abundantly in the area. The Spanish followed this advice and were thus able to keep their horses well nourished and restore their normal fertility. The Spanish were deeply impressed.

The Spanish found strong, healthy babies and adults in the hostile highlands, a condition attributable to a diet consisting mostly of maca. The Inca, and subsequently the Spanish, used maca as a staple food and fed it to livestock. It didn't take long for the Spanish to figure out that whatever was in maca that enhanced animal fertility might promote sexual benefits in humans as well. The Inca considered maca to be a gift from the gods, along with potatoes and corn. The Spanish, plunderers of all Incan riches, discovered in maca a worthy aphrodisiac.

Today maca is becoming increasingly popular in Peru among native and nonnative people, and the effects of maca are creating market demand in Japan, Europe, and the United States. Maca cultivation is on the increase just as Professor Cardenas predicted, a number of government experts and agencies are actively promoting maca agriculture and development, and maca is becoming a major botanical product on the international herbal scene.

Maca's Inner Secrets

Maca is a nutritious food. Dried maca contains about 59 percent carbohydrate and has a protein value of slightly more than 10 percent. It possesses a higher lipid content than other root crops at 2.2 percent, of which linoleic acid, palmitic acid, and oleic acid are the primary fatty acids. Maca is also a rich source of sterols, including sitosterol, campestrol, ergosterol, brassicasterol, and ergostadienol. Maca also possesses a good amount of iron, potassium, and calcium.

What agents in maca are responsible for its potent sex-enhancing effects? The plant sterols listed may possibly be some of the chemical agents of desire, as may be isothiocyanates discovered in the root. Though these compounds occur in small amounts, they may enhance fertility. Two other groups of compounds, recently discovered, appear to be the sexual keys to this high-altitude root.

At PureWorld Botanicals, Dr. Qun Yi Zheng and his team of analytical chemists dissected maca root from a chemical standpoint, utilizing the most sophisticated technology available today. Dr. Zheng and his partners discovered two previously unknown groups of novel compounds in maca, the macamides and macaenes. And though these compounds occur in very small quantities, their effect is significant. Experiments with animals show these two groups of compounds to be very powerful sex and energy enhancers. In the experiments, frequency of copulation and stamina increased radically as the quantities of macamides and macaenes in the diet increased.

Discovering the activity of new compounds in plants is not a complete process until the results are published in a peer-reviewed scientific journal. In April 2000, an article entitled, "Effect of a lipidic extract from *Lepidium meyenii* on sexual behavior in mice and rats," ran in the medical journal *Urology*. In the article, Dr. Zheng and his colleagues described experiments in which increased doses of the macamides and macaenes resulted in greatly increased sexual activity among the animals studied.

Yet another article on the stamina-enhancing effects of maca extract appeared in the American Chemical Society proceedings in 2002. In this article, Zheng and colleagues reported increased stamina in animals given the proprietary extract of maca manufactured by PureWorld, MacaPure. Use of maca significantly improved stamina in animals studied.

Following the science conducted at PureWorld, Dr. Michael Balick of the New York Botanical Garden and Dr. Roberta Lee, M.D., wrote a feature for *Alternative Therapies* magazine entitled, "Maca: from traditional food to energy and libido stimulant." In the paper, the two authors described the path that maca has taken to arrive in the present as a scientifically established sex enhancer. Toward the end of the article, the authors quoted PureWorld's president Natalie Koether, the person who directed me to head to Peru. When asked if maca was being positioned as a natural Viagra, she said, "Not so much as that it acts more on the libido, whereas Viagra acts more on mechanical function. Response to the extracts of maca has been terrific, and while men report it works, we have also gotten some good feedback from a physician who uses it with success for menopausal women."

As it turned out, PureWorld became the leading company in

the maca extract field. As a result of scientific advancement and high-quality source material, PureWorld developed MacaPure, which contains 0.6 percent macamides and macaenes. This is the only standardized extract of maca, which was used in the studies described above. This is how a traditional plant remedy develops into a botanical product in a nontraditional market. In the case of maca, the standardized extract MacaPure enables people to derive the sexual benefits of maca at a far smaller dose than the powdered root. The extract promotes overall energy and stamina, and significantly boosts libido and sexual function in both men and women.

A Maca Jamboree

Sergio, his friend Enriqué, and I jammed ourselves into the Toyota with all our gear and set off for the Central Highlands to Cerro de Pasco, about a nine-hour drive. Our mission was to see a number of people involved in maca agriculture and commerce. Heading east from the arid desert land around Lima, we cruised to higher elevation, mostly on narrow two-lane paved roads. As we moved up, the air grew cooler, the hillsides around us got higher, the drops off the sides of the road fell farther down, and the switchbacks that zigged and zagged up into the mountains became steeper. Mining trucks and buses roared around blind corners. In some places, large rockslides narrowed the road. The sky was overcast for almost the whole ride, a blanket of gray over the landscape. It seemed poor weather for spring.

As we wound our way around the mountains and climbed higher, we traversed great grassy valleys that stretched for dozens of miles, many of which afforded spectacular views of high, snow-capped Andean peaks. At hundreds of places, horsetail waterfalls cascaded down steep, rocky slopes, rushing into ravines, surging rapidly toward lower elevations. Bubbling springs flowed from fissures in rocks at high elevations, creating a world of streams, brooks, waterfalls, bubbling cascades, vigorous rivers, and rivulets, all seeking lower ground. In some places, streams rushed right across the road. As we got higher up in the mountains, snow began to fall, heavy and wet, slowing our progress and reducing visibility. At the highest point on our trip we were at over sixteen thousand feet. After nine hours of hard riding we pulled into Cerro de Pasco, the center of maca commerce in the highlands.

Cerro de Pasco is a grimy mining town with one of the largest open pit mines on earth. When we arrived, a noxious miasma covered the town in a cold cloud. Cerro de Pasco features the largest population, 65,000 people, living at the highest altitude anywhere in the world, at almost 4,575 meters (15,000 feet). Humble mud dwellings and tin shanties lined rutted, muddy streets and narrow alleys. But fortune favored us. We learned that in just two days, Cerro de Pasco would host the Third Annual National Maca Festival. The coincidental timing of our visit to Cerro and the festival was pure serendipity.

Two mornings after our arrival, a grassy fairground in Cerro was transformed into a bustling enclave of tents, tarps, tabletops, and displays of every conceivable aspect of maca cultivation and processing. Several booths displayed the many colors of maca roots. A few exhibited broad, seed-bearing maca flowers, and some maca growers demonstrated how the seeds are shaken from their pods, then screened and cleaned, yielding maca seed for the next year's planting. A few maca growers displayed healthy maca plants in small ceramic pots. The growers were surprised to see me especially, and asked Sergio and Enrique why we were there. We explained that maca was likely to become popular in the United States, and we wanted to see as much of the local maca scene as possible. All the growers we met seemed to take our interest as a positive sign.

Across the grassy park from the agricultural displays, booths and tables displayed maca food products of all types. One man stood beside a large display of nicely packaged maca cookies. "Are they any good?" I inquired. He offered me a cookie that tasted much like a well-made graham cracker, but denser and crunchier. At several booths, women busily cranked out maca blender drinks. The typical shake included a couple of soaked maca roots and a little bit of the soaking water, a handful of fresh papaya trucked up from the warm lowlands, some condensed milk, an egg, honey, and vanilla. Tasting one blender drink meant being obliged to taste them all, so as not to offend anybody. We stopped at six or seven booths, sampling the blender drinks made at each one. Along the way, I shot still photographs. The women making the blender drinks were proud to be photographed with their ingredients and appliances. I asked each one of them why people drank maca shakes. They all smiled, a few laughed, and the answer was uniform—energy and sex. Great sex, to be exact.

At one booth I encountered a large, simmering pot of *mazzamora*, a porridge made of maca, the Andean grains quinoa and kiwicha, eggs, milk, honey, and vanilla. This, the woman behind the counter told me, is eaten by many people each morning. "You will notice the effect of this breakfast," she told me as she offered a bowl. The porridge was really good. We also came upon maca "Jell-O" and maca flan. Both were surprisingly good tasting, though I favored the flan. Several women made maca marmalade, which they sold in small plastic tubs. At one booth, a man and woman produced maca chips in a little fry-olator as fast as they could, and people were eating them up twice as quickly.

We discovered several kinds of bottled maca products at the festival as well, including sweet maca syrup, bottled juices with maca, and maca liquor. Every maker of maca liquor assured us that theirs was the very best and plied us with drinks to prove it. The maca liquor tasted nutty and delicious and exerted an especially potent effect in the thin high atmosphere. I felt loopy on the alcohol in the thin air.

Throughout the entire festival, Sergio and Enrique and I talked with vendors and sampled all the maca products—I found myself keyed up from all the maca. I asked more than a hundred people why they ate maca, drank maca, or used it in any of its forms. "They're all going to tell you the same thing," Sergio commented. It was true, everybody mentioned sex and energy.

Physicians and Maca

The use of maca for sexual and reproductive purposes is not just limited to the cookie and flan market. The plant is pre-scribed in Peruvian medical practices as well. Hugo Malaspina, M.D., a cardiologist practicing complementary medicine in Lima, has been using maca in his practice for more than a dozen years, and commonly recommends maca to women experienc-ing premenstrual discomfort or menopausal symptoms. "There are different medicinal plants that work on the ovaries by stim-ulating them. With maca though, we should say that it regulates the ovarian function." Dr. Malaspina further commented that

"Maca regulates the organs of internal secretion, such as the pituitary, the adrenal glands, the pancreas, etc. I have had perhaps two hundred female patients whose perimenopausal and menopausal symptoms are alleviated by taking maca."

Aguila Calderon, M.D., is the former dean of the Faculty of Human Medicine at the National University of Federico Villarreal in Lima. In his medical practice, Dr. Calderon prescribes maca for male impotence, erectile dysfunction, menopausal symptoms, and general fatigue. "Maca has a lot of easily absorbable calcium in it, plus magnesium, and a fair amount of silica which we are finding very useful in treating the decalcification of bones in children and adults."

A number of holistic and complementary medical doctors in the United States, from general practitioners to psychiatrists, are using maca with a variety of patients. Menopausal women experience relief from various uncomfortable symptoms of menopause. Both men and women report a significant boost in libido, and a number of men who have suffered from erectile dysfunction have improved, as a result of taking maca. One New York psychiatrist I know recommends maca to those who take Prozac. That antidepressant often sends libido plummeting, and he finds that maca brings it back. It takes many years to inculcate a plant medicine into a large number of medical practices, but with maca this process is happening.

The Shaman's Storm

In the evening after the maca festival, Sergio, Enriqué, three men involved with maca agriculture, and I piled into the Toyota and another pickup truck and headed out of Cerro de Pasco to Ninagaga, a small highland town where Sergio had purchased land to build a maca center. Enriqué planned to perform a shamanic purification ritual to bless the land, and to invoke the blessings of the spirits. "Then that place will be very lively and protected," he said. By the time we arrived in Ninagaga, the sun was setting and a cold wind was blowing hard through the highlands. In the center of Sergio's field, Enriqué piled together a shin-high pile of twigs and boards for a fire, which we set aflame. When the fire was lit, Enriqué set up an altar on the ground, replete with artifacts of various kinds, including a small wooden sword, some polished sticks, crystals, a ceramic pyramid, a woven medicine bag, a small satchel of coca leaves, and figurines of deities from the Christian, Hindu, Buddhist, and Egyptian traditions.

As Enriqué prepared for the ceremony, two strange men came across the field toward us. The men looked briefly at our pitifully small fire and slipped away after a few muttered words. A few moments later they returned with huge armloads of freshly cut straw, which they added to the fire. The fire crackled and sprang high with leaping flames. The two men slipped off into the darkness, and we never saw them again.

Enriqué opened a bottle of high-octane cane alcohol called *pisco* and poured a small amount in a cup. He drank some and threw some at the fire as he chanted softly to himself. Enriqué removed his jacket and rolled up his shirtsleeves. He appeared to be sweating. The rest of us were shivering cold against a bitter wind and gathered as close to the fire as possible. Enriqué began to chant, calling out to the gods and spirits. He chewed a large quid of coca leaf and splashed a lot of *pisco* around. Then he produced a well-tied package about the size of a loaf of bread and placed it in the fire. He poured more *pisco*, drank some, sprinkled some on the fire, and splashed some more around. As the package burned, Enriqué waved his arms about and called to the spirits. Black, ominous clouds roiled overhead, thunder boomed and lightning flashed in sky-splitting streaks.

When the package was fairly well burned, Enriqué poured some amber crystals onto the fire. The crystals sparked and the aroma rose like pungent church incense. Enriqué spoke to each person in the group, giving specific insights and extending wishes for blessings from the spirits. "May this place be protected and sacred, may the maca give life to many, and may the mission of the people here remain pure." When he was finished, he put some more straw on the fire, splashed some more *pisco* around and drank some more, and declared the purification ritual for the Ninagaga maca center complete. At the exact moment that Enriqué declared the finish of the ceremony, the sky boomed with bomblike thunder, the wind rose to a howling, and a driving rain raged down upon us. We ran yelling in the dark back to our trucks.

Using Maca

Many supplement companies who are selling maca are putting about 500 milligrams of ground dried maca in each capsule. I believe that to garner any benefit from maca you would have to take a minimum of ten 500 milligram capsules of powdered maca daily, equal to five grams of maca. You can certainly take more. Remember that maca is a food. It produces a very powerful sexual effect, but it will not do so in tiny quantities. If you are using powdered maca root in a capsule, you need to take a lot.

MacaPure, a standardized extract of maca, is more concentrated. The extract contains a specific concentration of macamides and macaenes, the particular compounds in maca that have been found to enhance sexual activity in tests with animals. I would say that MacaPure will give very significant results at a dose of 1,000–2,000 milligrams (1–2 grams) per day. Savvy companies state that they use MacaPure on their product labels, mostly for encapsulated supplements.

Powdered maca root is also available in natural food stores. If you make blender drinks with powdered maca, throw in a tablespoon. The more maca or maca extract you consume, the more benefit you are likely to get. In toxicity studies conducted in the United States, maca showed absolutely no toxicity and no adverse pharmacologic effects. In animal studies, the more maca animals consume, the stronger and more sexually active they become. You can be generous with the amounts of maca products you take.

TAO OF SEX

Siberian Ginseng and Red Ginseng

IN THE UNITED STATES, WHEN SOMEBODY SAYS THEY'RE TAKing you to a health food restaurant, you basically know what you're getting into. The menu will feature a few salads, soups, various grain and bean dishes, tofu entrees, fresh-squeezed juices, carrot cake, herbal teas. But it's all different in China. Seated in a private room at a Beijing health food restaurant, I watched with great fascination as one strange dish after another was set down before our group. Bright silk lamps hung over our circular table. Murals on the wall depicted Taoist mountain scenes with craggy landscapes. Angular banjos played moody Chinese music on discreet speakers. Three silk-clad women hovered nearby, making sure that we wanted for nothing and our glasses were full.

As soon as the rice balls hit the table, my friend Gordon was on them with chopsticks. He was apparently very hungry. I ate a couple myself and watched with amusement as he chowed down one rice ball after another in rapid succession. "Man, these little sesame-covered rice balls are great," he declared with relish in a brief pause between chews. I leaned close.

"Gordon, when was the last time you saw sesame seeds with antennae?" He looked horrified. "Those are small black ants, buddy." And so the meal went like that, with ant-covered rice balls, a viscious gray wild mountain frog stew, a fragrant worm salad, herb-glazed rabbit, black snails, chicken and chiles, lotus root, several dark sauces, a steaming soup of wild mushrooms and woody roots, various small plates of fungus, candied red ginseng slices, fish, scallops, spicy cabbage, nutted pork, herbal tea, beer, rice wine, and the pièce de résistance, a heaping platter of fried scorpions. When the scorpions arrived, Gordon cast an alarmed glance my way. I took the only reasonable course of action under the circumstances. Deftly snatching a big scorpion with my sticks, I popped it into my mouth, chewed thoughtfully for a moment, and pronounced "not bad" to the table. In fact, it tasted like a potato chip. It was one of the most remarkable and bizarre meals I have ever enjoyed.

My friends Gordon and Xiao Nan Gray run a business called China Liaisons and had made various contacts for our trip to the Chinese capital of Beijing and to the very far northeast to Harbin. Our mission was to investigate the manufacturing and use of both Siberian ginseng (*Eleutherococcus senticosus*) and Red ginseng (*Panax ginseng*). As two of China's most powerful vitality-enhancing herbs, both were of great commercial interest to us. As two legendary hot plants, both were of special interest to me. At the health food restaurant in Beijing, we were hosted by a senior trade official named Mr. Shen, who was delighted that we enjoyed the hospitality. He wanted to make sure we understood that we were partaking of a brilliantly devised combination of tonics and elixirs designed to bestow health and vigor. "You see," he told us, "every dish has special herbs and medicinal agents, all designed to balance the five elements in your system and establish a perfect balance of yin and yang."

In Traditional Chinese Medicine, or TCM, beneficial foods, beverages, and herbs are employed to enhance harmony among the five primary life-forces within us, known as the "five elements": earth, water, fire, wood, and air. Our dinner represented just the right combination of ingredients, skillfully concocted in the kitchen, designed to set us in a natural state of harmony. This, we were told, would then establish a balance of yin and yang, the polarities within all things. Achieving a perfect balance of yin and yang is tantamount to achieving a state of grace. It was a lofty goal for a long dinner.

I was impressed by Mr. Shen's informed description of the numerous herbs and fungus in our meal. The sauces and broths included a number of tonic herbs. These botanical treasures are used to enhance overall health and vitality and are employed in the treatment of various disorders, notably fatigue, stress, anxiety, sleeplessness, weakness, or susceptibility to common ailments. The various species of fungus we ate help to boost overall immunity, detoxify the body, improve cardiovascular function, kill viruses, and promote vitality. I listened keenly at the mention of both wucha and Red ginseng. "These two herbs, you know them," Mr. Shen told us. "They are treasure to us, because they build basic life-force. They are in a special class of all herbs. They are at the top."

Black Dragon River

The farthest northeastern province in China, Heilongjiang occupies much of the region formerly known as Manchuria. The province takes its name from the Amur River, known to the Chinese as the "Black Dragon River," which marks the boundary between China and Siberia. Heilongjiang covers an area of more than 460,000 square kilometers, bordering Mongolia to the west, and Russia on the northeast.

I awoke before dawn in the Hou Auan Cun (Garden Hamlet) Hotel in the sprawling Soviet-style city of Harbin, the administrative center of Heilongjiang province. Chairman Mao, I was told, used to stay in the hotel. The low, private building was a favorite of the Politburo. A high wall surrounded the grounds, a gatehouse stood at the only entrance, and armed guards patrolled the perimeter. The security was overdone, but did provide employment. My cavernous room could have accommodated a large family, and I could have played racketball in the tiled bathroom. Heavy green drapes hung over high, wide windows. Laminate was peeling off the woodwork. The carpet was stained from one end to the other with decades of tobacco spit. It was strange.

In winter, Harbin offers months of subzero temperatures and is known as "Ice City." In May the climate was pleasant. I dressed, grabbed my camera and several rolls of film, and headed out to find a morning market. There had to be one. Within about twenty minutes, I was walking through a crowded outdoor market of vegetables, fruits, meats, fish, grains, beans, eggs, dry goods of all types, knockoffs of every known brand, and herbs, stall after stall of herbs. The place bustled with lively activity. I did not speak Mandarin, and nobody near me seemed to speak English. When I walked up to one herb stand and said, "Wucha," the man behind the table nodded, smiled, and pointed to a pile of roots.

"I would rather have a handful of wucha than a cartload of

gold and jewels," wrote the famous Chinese herbalist Li Shi-Chen in his 1596 treatise on herbal medicine *Ben Cao Gang Mu*. First discussed as a valuable medicine over 2,000 years ago in the herbal treatise *The Divine Husbandman's Classic of the Materia Medica,* wucha refers to the roots of *Eleutherococcus senticosus,* a plant which grows wild in abundance in the Xiaoxinganling Mountains of Heilongjiang Province. In the United States, wucha is commonly sold as "Siberian ginseng," though it not a true ginseng species. Though the plant does belong to the same family, Araliaceae, wucha owes its popular Siberian ginseng name to its ginsenglike properties and effects. Legislation passed in the United States now prohibits wucha, or "Eleuthero" from being labeled Siberian ginseng. Despite the confusion over its name, wucha, or Siberian ginseng, or *Eleutherococcus senticosus,* is an extraordinary herb that strengthens the body, enhances performance, and gives a tremendous boost to sexual vigor and function.

A shrub that grows as high as nine feet, *Eleutherococcus senticosus* reaches maturity in seven or more years. The plant grows throughout northeast Asia, in parts of Russia, China, Korea, and Japan, but it is most abundant in Heilongjiang, where it is common undergrowth in forests and sometimes grows in great, impenetrable thickets. The plant yields a woody root that is one of the most highly prized medicinal plants in the vast Chinese herbal pharmacopoeia. Employed in Traditional Chinese Medicine to invigorate sexual function, boost vital energy, and normalize body functions, wucha is classified as an adaptogen, enhancing immunity and vitality overall. It is considered an exceptionally valuable tonic with broad uses and benefits.

Later in the morning of my market meander, Gordon, Xiao Nan, and I arrived at the Heilongjiang Institute of Traditional

Chinese Medicine. I had been advised to go there by my old friend Alex Anatole, who used to be in the KGB and knew a lot about Manchuria. His suggestion was a fortunate tip. The institute, as it turned out, was the foremost center in China for research into wucha. Over the course of a few decades, the institute had culled material from ancient herbal texts and then set out to determine the veracity of traditional health claims made for the plant. In many studies, the Heilongjiang Institute of Traditional Chinese Medicine had found that consumption of wucha enhances immunity, increases strength, stimulates sexual function, improves sleep, helps the body during times of oxygen deprivation, enhances cardiovascular function, improves athletic performance, and sharpens mental alertness.

The Root: Wucha's Treasure

At the institute, we met with Dr. Xiao, one of the directors of research. He explained to us the significance of wucha. "It is not usual at all for one plant to do so much. Most of the time, if you investigate the health properties of a plant, you will find that it does just a few things well. But with wucha, we see that it is like a life plant. It helps everybody and is very safe. It will help almost every condition, and it builds vitality." Dr. Xiao described that wucha, as an adaptogen, helped to build great strength and vitality. "For this reason, it was regarded as treasure by the ancient sages. Now we understand that this was not just a quaint notion. They understood the power of the plant very well." What about the sexual effects of wucha, I asked. "For sex, wucha is comparable to ginseng, and is better than almost any other herb in traditional Chinese medicine. Wucha has the power to build up sexual vitality a great deal. And so it helps to slow down sexual aging, and to restore sexual ability if there are problems."

Generous with his time, Dr. Xiao took us on a tour of the institute facilities, which included a small lab, a modest library, and an herbarium with voucher samples of plants, most notable *Eleutherococcus senticosus*. "We keep specimens of wucha here, so if any scientist in any other place needs a valid specimen, we can provide that."

Dr. Xiao told us that scientists at the institute as well as in Russia have found numerous active substances in wucha, including sterols, coumarins, flavonoids, and polysaccharides. Some of the specific compounds in wucha that have been isolated for research include daucosterol, syringaresinol, isofraxidin, hyperine, sesamin, friedelin, and syringin. Like *Rhodiola rosea*, ashwagandha, and ginseng, wucha is classified as an adaptogen, enhancing immunity to a wide variety of adverse health influences. This effect is believed to be due to its concentration of a family of compounds known as eleutherosides, but the mechanisms by which wucha functions as an adaptogen remain unknown.

Despite the lack of a thorough understanding of wucha's adaptogenic powers, a few things are known with respect to its specific immune-enhancing effects. Two polysaccharides in wucha display specific immune-enhancing power by promoting phagocytosis (the means by which protective cells engulf harmful microorganisms, damaged cells, and foreign particles), and the promotion of protective B lymphocytes, which are protective agents manufactured by the immune system. Further studies show that wucha helps to defend the body against some bacterial and chemical toxins.

Pharmacological evaluation conducted in both China and

Russia on the various compounds in Wucha have determined that Wucha's stimulation of sexual and adrenal functions is due to its various sterols; its sedative activity is attributable to coumarins; its beneficial effects upon the cardiovascular system are due to flavonoids; and its antitumor activity is an effect of polysaccharides. Listed in the *Chinese Pharmacopoeia,* wucha is one of the best-documented plants in herbal medicine and has been used traditionally and clinically in the treatment of cancer, leukocytopenia, hypertension, hypotension, atherosclerosis, nervous fatigue, and other diseases.

Studies of wucha's effects on human performance conducted in both Russia and China show that wucha increases human tolerance to a broad range of stress factors, including heat, noise, and increased exercise. When taken regularly, wucha increases work output, endurance, athletic performance, and mental alertness. Wucha also shows remarkable protective benefits under conditions of serious oxygen deprivation. Due to its stress-reducing and extraordinary performance-enhancing powers, wucha is popular among factory workers, athletes, miners, soldiers, deep-sea divers, and others who engage in physically and mentally demanding tasks and occupations. The effect of the plant upon sexual function is almost taken for granted. In cases of sexual fatigue, wucha restores vigor. In cases of impotence, wucha restores erectile function. The root boosts desire in both men and women. It is widely used as a tonic, in tea and also in small glass ampules filled with extract.

On the way back into the city from the institute, Gordon and Xiao-Nan and I stopped to admire a small thicket of *Eleutherococcus senticosus* plants growing near the roadside. We were well aware of the wide distribution of the plant, since Dr. Xiao had shown us a map that identified large areas of wucha. I am always thrilled to see high-value medicinal plants in the wild, and was grateful to see wucha in its native habitat. Over the course of our time in Harbin, as we traveled from one place to another, we would see many stands of wild wucha.

Harbin #1

On the outskirts of the city, we arrived at Harbin Pharmaceutical Factory #1. The long and low concrete building sat amid a great surrounding expanse of open undeveloped land. The facility reminded me of an army camp. Inside, we were greeted warmly by the director Mr. Zhang and his assistant Mae. "Thank you for coming here," Mr. Zhang told us. "We do not receive many visitors from the United States, so we are pleased that you have come to see us." With that greeting, we were taken upstairs to an open conference room where tea and biscuits waited for us on a low table. Several other managers from the factory joined us, and we explained our interest in their wucha products.

Mr. Zhang led us to a display case in the hall near the conference room, where every product manufactured at Harbin #1 was displayed with medals of achievement and certificates of outstanding quality. While we admired the dozens of products in the case, Mr. Zhang instructed Mae to bring some samples into the conference room. Shortly after being reseated, Mae came in with a large tray of wucha samples. Among them were single-serve glass ampules of pure wucha, wucha with royal jelly, wucha with deer antler. We were also shown wucha in soluble granules, and a thick, concentrated wucha paste extract. After surveying the samples, I said that I would like to try them, to appreciate their flavor and effect. A large dispenser of hot water, numerous cups, spoons, and small plates were brought to the table. "You should please try these, to see for yourself our quality," advised Liu, one of the managers.

More than a dozen products of various sizes, concentrations, and forms were opened and prepared for my consideration. After I drank each one, I was expected to make comment, so I remarked on flavor or sweetness or some other attribute. As the next two hours wore on, I felt a deep, strong, very potent energy welling up inside me. By the time the sampling session was through, I had consumed more wucha than I typically used in half a year.

I recall a time once when I ordered an herbal elixir at Tee-garden's Herbal Emporium in Venice, California. The drink, called a Reverend Michael, was billed as especially invigorating. As the woman who made the concoction served me she said, "I hope you have a date tonight." It was a great line, and I never forgot it. At the end of our time at Harbin #1, I wished very much that I had a date that night. Alas, I did not.

How Much Wucha

If you take wucha by any name, whether as wucha, Eleuthero, or Siberian ginseng, you have choices. If you are taking a capsule or tablet, look for one that contains a concentrated extract of wucha. A daily dose of 500–1,000 milligrams should impart the benefits of the plant. Even better, look for a concentrated black "paste" extract of wucha and drink one to two cups of tea, each made with a pea-sized blob of the extract, twice daily. Or obtain ampules of wucha extract and consume one to three per day. Wucha delivers a strong energetic and strengthening vitality and definitely makes you want to have a date tonight.

Markets of Hong Kong

Walking along Queensway in Hong Kong in the sweltering heat and humidity of June, I passed meat shops featuring hanging ducks, bakeries displaying round bean-filled doughnuts, vegetable stands with durian—the most smelly fruit on earth, fabric shops displaying brilliant silks, and several herbal shops. Just standing outside in front of the herb shops, I could smell woody and sweet aromas, a complex fragrance of healing power. Of all the medicinal plants displayed in the shops, ginseng root (*Panax ginseng*) was consistently most prominent. Ginseng roots were offered in heaping piles and display cases featured dozens of roots large and small. This came as no surprise.

Ginseng is so legendary that almost everyone has at least heard of it. Regarded as a supreme tonic herb in traditional Chinese medicine, ginseng stimulates the central nervous system, invigorates the brain, increases resistance to stress and fatigue, and sharpens the mind. Ginseng is also an adaptogen, an agent that enhances general immune resistance. It is used by athletes to enhance strength and endurance and to help improve coordination. In animal studies, ginseng increases sexual activity, and millions of human users swear by this plant to enhance libido and sexual vitality. In my estimation, ginseng is one of the most beneficial plants in nature. It enhances vitality and is definitely an important part of any good antiaging regime.

In the Hong Kong herbal shops, I admired the various sizes

of ginseng roots and selected several red roots for my own pleasure. A couple of stores offered free ginseng tea, and I helped myself to a cup at each one. The tea was stimulating and helped me to shake off the fatigue resulting from the oppressive heat. I had used ginseng almost daily for decades and was pleased to acquire high-quality roots at reasonable prices. Like wucha, ginseng is native to northeast China, Korea, and Russia. This slow-growing perennial takes about six years to produce a mature root, which is probably the single most widely used medicinal herb on earth. When harvested, the root is a beige color, but many ginseng roots undergo an alchemical process, including steaming and infusion with other herbs, resulting in "red" ginseng. No ginseng grows red. It is an herbal preparation, a special curing secret process guarded jealously.

Ginseng's name *Panax ginseng* sort of says it all. *Panax* is derived from the Greek *pan,* which means all, and *akos,* meaning cure. Though ginseng is no panacea, it is useful for restoring health and vitality in hundreds of ailments. Like wucha, ginseng was first described in the 2,000-year-old text *Shen Nong Cao Jing*. The root is used primarily to build vitality and is listed in the national pharmacopoeias of France, Germany, Austria, Switzerland, China, Japan, and Russia.

Ginseng has been the subject of many human clinical studies. The root appears to protect against various forms of cancer, to help stabilize blood sugar in people with non-insulin-dependent diabetes, to boost immune function, to reduce high blood pressure, to improve quality of life under stress, to enhance performance during exercise, to improve erectile function, and to increase male fertility. Ginseng root helps to allay fatigue and improve overall physical and mental performance.

Ginseng has had its detractors over time, who have emphatically insisted that the root doesn't provide any sexual enhancement at all. That notion was neatly dispelled by a study of forty-five men with an average age of fifty-four. In the placebo-controlled, double-blind study, neither the researchers nor the subjects knew what they were taking. Half the group consumed 900 milligrams of red ginseng root per day and the other half consumed a placebo. The results? Those who consumed the ginseng root experienced a 42 percent improvement in erectile function. Researchers speculate that ginseng improves erectile function by increasing nitric oxide in the penis, dilating the vessels of the corpus cavernosum. This is the same mechanism by which Viagra works. Ginseng is appreciably safer than Viagra, which can cause serious side effects. Ginseng is also appreciably less expensive.

A Happy Recipe

Now I am going to let you in on a secret, a way to derive maximum benefit from ginseng for a very modest cost. Ginseng is one of the more expensive herbs for its weight, because the root takes a long time to mature. Part of the cost of ginseng also has to do with its great value to health. Ginseng root contains a class of compounds called ginsenosides. These compounds produce the numerous benefits of ginseng and are concentrated in the root.

There are two parts to ginseng root. The main root is what you will find in most stores. But attached to the main root upon harvest are finer "hairs," or "tailings." The tailings are the parts most concentrated with the ginsenosides. Though the ginsenosides are of enormous value to human health, the ginseng plant doesn't accumulate those compounds for our purposes. The plant contains ginsenosides to help ward off invasion and rot due to microorganisms in soil. The ginsenosides, like many compounds in plants, help to protect the ginseng plant itself.

Once or twice every year, I make a trip to a Chinese grocery or herbal shop to pick up one or two big bags of red ginseng tailings. I stop to admire the whole red roots, which may cost as much as twenty dollars for just an ounce or two. Then I purchase one or two pounds of even more highly concentrated tailings for about twelve dollars per pound. The savings are significant. At home, I fill a mason jar to the top with the ginseng talings. Then I pour pure vodka into the jar, until the vodka comes all the way up to the top.

Vodka makes an excellent extraction solvent: it is clean and readily available. After filling the mason jar with ginseng tailings and vodka, I cap the jar and let it sit for a month or so. Every day I give the jar a little shake, turning it upside down and then right side up again. After a month, the extract is ready to use. I take a teaspoon of the extract with a couple of ounces of water, and get a far more concentrated ginseng than I would derive from most products available on the shelf.

Ginseng is a healthful plant tonic with thousands of years of safe and effective use. But even regular ginseng users often do not take enough to experience ginseng's palpable benefits. If you take enough ginseng, you will feel it. When I use my homemade extract, I notice an immediate feeling of energy, strength, and stamina. And don't worry about the vodka, unless you are an alcoholic. In that case, never use an alcohol extract of anything. Otherwise, a teaspoon of vodka-infused ginseng extract contains a small amount of alcohol. In winter, when it is freezing outside, I take two teaspoons of my home-made extract. The effect is bracing, and it helps me to deal with the cold.

Using Ginseng

First and foremost, I recommend my homemade extract but many of you who read this book will prefer tablets and cap-sules. In that case, look for products that are made with an ex-tract of ginseng standardized to 4 percent or more ginsenosides. Take about 500 milligrams of such a product, and you will derive benefits. Also, you will find a number of single dose gin-seng ampule products available. Those ampules usually con-tain about 500 milligrams of ginseng. One or more of the ampules daily will give you a good effect. Like wucha, ginseng is also available in a thick black paste extract. A pea-sized blob of paste extract in a cup of hot water once or twice daily will give you a noticeable ginseng effect.

Ginseng is one of nature's wonder plants. If you like, you can eat roots or tailings. I remember a time back in 1972 when a group of my friends and I were driving home to Massachu-setts from the West Coast. Before heading back, we stopped in San Francisco's Chinatown and loaded up on herbs. I pur-chased a bag of ginseng roots and munched on them while driving. By the time we reached Indiana, I was so stimulated by the ginseng, I did not want to relinquish the wheel. I drove straight through until pulling into the driveway at home. The ginseng made me highly alert, focused, and definitely ready to drive. Though I am not recommending that you consume as much ginseng as I did on that trip, I can tell you that it made me feel great, and the ride home passed pleasantly.

Here is another tip for you. Make ginseng tea for yourself and your partner before making love. I do not recommend the granular tea mixes that come in packets, because they are about 85 percent. Instead, make tea either with paste extract or with tailings. Enjoy the lift.

THE LOVE DRUG

Chocolate

PEOPLE HAVE LONG TURNED TO CHOCOLATE TO ADD EXTRA sensuous dimension and pleasure to lovemaking. Chocolate is made from the seeds, known as cocoa beans, of the tropical tree *Theobroma cacao*. The Aztec Emperor Montezuma II reputedly drank a large goblet of frothy, unsweetened chocolate prior to bedding the women in his harem. Being emperor had its privileges, and Montezuma enjoyed the finest chocolate in his empire and the intimate company of the fairest young maidens as well. In 1519, Spanish plunderer Hernán Cortés landed at Tabasco on Mexico's Gulf of Campeche and was mistaken by Montezuma and his people as the returned tenth-century Toltec ruler Topiltzin Quetzalcoatl, whose status over time had been upgraded to that of a god. Montezuma gave up his throne to Cortés with these words: "Welcome to you, our master, on your return to your country among your own people, to sit on your throne."

Cortés was showered with gifts, including groaning sacks of cocoa beans, which served as the currency of the realm. The Aztec prepared a delicious and refreshing drink of finely ground cocoa beans, mixed in water and beaten to a froth with a wooden stirring instrument called a molinet. The Aztecs called chocolate *cacahuatl,* and the drink was for the privileged. People of high social standing, including members of the royal house, nobility, and warriors, drank *cacahuatl*. Emperor Montezuma reputedly consumed as many as fifty large frothy cups of the drink daily.

Columbus, seventeen years before, had also been given cocoa beans, though not because he was mistaken for a god. The Genoese explorer apparently drank the native frothy chocolate beverage, finding it bitter and spicy. Columbus paid no further notice to the beans he was given. By the time he died four years later, nothing had come of his brush with chocolate, the use of which predated the Aztecs. Cortés, on the other hand, recognized chocolate as a New World delicacy of potentially great economic value.

Sometime around 1000 B.C. the Olmec, who were early Mayans, are believed to have cultivated the cacao tree for the first time. The Mayan civilization flourished from the Yucatan Peninsula to the Pacific Coast of Guatemala. The Maya called the delicious and mood-enhancing product made from the beans of the cacao tree *tchocolatl*. The Maya believed that the god of all creation, known as "Heart of Sky," had fashioned the first humans out of water and earth and wood and maize and cacao and various fruits. To the Maya, chocolate was not just a marvelous food; it was an agent of the divine, an essential part of human beings. Use of chocolate spread to the Aztec civilization. The Aztecs introduced Hernán Cortés to the product whose name *Theobroma* means food of the gods.

Realizing there was a great deal of money to be made from the Aztec's vast cacao plantations, Cortés brought chocolate back to the Old World, where Europeans took it up with ardent enthusiasm. Chocolate can be considered one of the most enduring products of all time, a titan of international commerce and the preferred gift of lovers, especially from men to women. For chocolate engenders sweet and sensuous feelings and infuses the user with a sense of love.

You could make the claim that chocolate is an aphrodisiac by virtue of smell, taste, and feel alone. Chocolate's rich flavor, silky mouth feel, and earthy aroma seduce the palate and tantalize the imagination. One chocolate aficionado was the legendary Venetian adventurer and author Giovanni Giacomo Casanova, a man of great learning and refined taste. Living in the 1700s, Casanova devoted much of his life to travel, gambling, and seduction. Casanova's name became synonymous with sexual conquest. He was well informed about the love benefits of chocolate, which he reputedly consumed before making love with women.

Chocolate's Devotee

"I think that you could call chocolate a soft drug. I think that a lot of chocolate consumption is based on an individual's need to self-medicate. They feel a need to have a certain amount of chemicals in their brain soup, in their cranium, and chocolate does that." Sitting with chocolatier Timothy Moley, I listened with rapt attention as he waxed effusive about the world's most popular love drug.

Timothy Moley is passionate and extremely knowledgeable about chocolate. If you are willing to sit and listen, he will offer a comprehensive and engaging discourse on the subject. "When I eat a piece of chocolate, I can taste the environment where the cacao was grown," he told me. "I taste the characteristics of the soil; I smell the environment. So for me, eating a piece of chocolate takes me to that place where the beans were grown. I enjoy chocolate on many levels. I enjoy the texture, I enjoy the complexity. Every batch is different. I enjoy the play of the flavors as they come out of the chocolate. It's a natural attraction for me. I like chocolate, and I like how I feel when I eat chocolate."

After spending many years in the herb and spice industry, Timothy applied his talent, discerning palate, and affinity for romance to producing the Chocolove brand of fine chocolates. Chocolove chocolates come in various strengths of cocoa content, including the brand's signature bar, the 70 percent cocoa Strong Dark. To promote the traditional use of chocolate as a gift of love, Timothy embossed a heart onto the label of each bar and includes a love poem inside each wrapper. Why give a dozen roses or a bottle of perfume, he argues, when you can give chocolate and score a direct hit Cupid style.

This is the reason that chocolate, above all other confections, has soared to dizzying heights of popularity and has been embraced by lovers around the world. Chocolate is not a sex enhancer per se. It is something finer—an agent of love itself. Some plants will produce a good erection or make you amorous. Chocolate is a substance of another order entirely. It promotes the actual love experience. Among all the plants and plant products on this great and vast planet, only chocolate does this.

Chocolate works its way into the human psyche in numerous ways. This beloved electuary conveys hundreds of natural compounds, many of which modify mood. In analytical laboratories, clinics, and research centers, chemists and physicians are discovering the means by which chocolate has earned its well-deserved name food of the gods. Both a mood food and a love drug, chocolate pleasantly alters your state of mind and tickles the heart chakra.

Hawaiian Bliss

Hernán Cortés landed at Tabasco, 481 years before I parked at the doorstep of The Original Hawaiian Chocolate Factory, in Keauhou, on the lush Kona coast of the big island of Hawaii. A modest-sized building stood surrounded by healthy cacao trees, many hanging with ripe red pods ready for harvest. Stepping inside with my friend Zachary Gibson, I watched two men wrestling with a heavy stainless-steel industrial mixing machine. One of the men looked up at us, sweat pouring from his brow, and introduced himself as Bob Cooper, owner of the chocolate factory. Bob extended a sticky hand in greeting, and then returned his attention to the mixer. He and his assistant grunted and strained for a couple of minutes, until the mixer rested in its exact correct place.

"Thanks for visiting us," Bob said. "We're just getting up and running here. We don't even have any chocolate to sell. We've still got some bugs to work out, but today is our first day of production. We've been building up to this for quite a while now. It's a pretty exciting day for us." As Bob explained himself, his assistant set a few plastic chocolate molds into place underneath a pipe from which rich, brown liquid chocolate slowly flowed. Zachary and I watched the fragrant chocolate running from the tap. The air in the little factory smelled of rich cocoa, fragrant flowers, and the Kona atmosphere. I wanted some of that chocolate. Bob realized we were distracted by the chocolate. He picked up a mold in which a couple of pieces of chocolate were cooling and handed one to each of us. "Here. Have some of our chocolate, fresh off the line. You guys are the first outsiders to try it." I popped the piece of chocolate into my mouth and succumbed to the delicious flavor and aroma.

"Oh, my god," I muttered. Bob gave the smile of a happy chef. The chocolate was stupendous, a smashing confectionery success, a rare delectable treat. "This is outrageous," I sputtered. Zachary didn't say anything at all; he was too busy laughing with pleasure.

"Pretty darn good, huh? Do you know that we're the only people in all of Hawaii making chocolate from Hawaiian cocoa beans? Nobody else is making real Hawaiian chocolate. There's nothing like it." The chocolate yielded a host of complex flavors, earthy and floral and rich and sweet and sensual. Yes, I said, it's wonderful. But I've seen a lot of chocolate around made in Hawaii. That was the catalytic comment that caused Bob Cooper to tell his story.

"You see a lot of so-called Hawaiian chocolate all over the place. But you know what? All that chocolate is made from African beans. I mean, there's nothing wrong with African beans, but it doesn't add up to Hawaiian chocolate. So what if the chocolate is made here? It's no different from Kona coffee. For years, coffee growers in Kona have been trying to protect their local brand. People all over the place have been calling coffee Kona when it comes from God knows where. Now, Kona coffee growers have a law to protect them. Only coffee grown on the Kona coast can be called Kona. I want the same thing with chocolate. Only Hawaiian grown and made chocolate should be called Hawaiian." When Zachary and I sympathized, he relaxed. "You two want to take a look around?" We said we'd love to.

Stepping outside of the sparkling new chocolate factory, Bob swept an arm at the land behind the building. "We have about thirteen hundred cacao trees here," he told us. "We don't make chocolate from any other source, just these trees. So you're never going to get African chcocolate coming out of our factory. Just pure Hawaiian."

The rain forest tree from which chocolate derives is *Theobroma cacao,* named by the eighteenth-century Swedish scientist Carl von Linne'. Botanical experts offer differing opinions regarding the origin of cacao. New genetic testing seems to have settled the matter, pointing to the Orinoco Valley of Venezuela as the first place where the tree grew. Wild cacao then presumably spread up into Mexico, where it was first cultivated. The tree ranges between four and eight meters in height, and its cinnamon brown trunk usually does not exceed two meters in length. The branches of the cacao tree are covered with shiny, dark green leaves about ten inches long and three inches wide. Though the tree bears fruit and flowers all year around, usually there are two harvest seasons for gathering the fruit. The actual months of harvest vary somewhat depending upon the location of the plantation.

Cacao trees bear large, distinctive, football-shaped fruit pods that jut out directly from the trunk and the lower branches. Young fruit pods tend to be greenish in color. As they mature over the course of five to six months, they become elliptical in shape and bright red or yellow in color. The fruit pods average about nine inches in length and typically contain thirty to forty almond-sized seeds (cocoa beans) nestled in a pale white flesh. These seeds are made into the heavenly food loved around the world, chocolate.

The three varieties of *Theobroma cacao* whose beans are used in the making of chocolate are *criollo, forastero,* and *trinitario.* Compared to the other two varieties, *criollo* cacao bears longer, pointed pods, with deep ridges and white seeds. *Criollo* is delicate and sensitive to variations in climate and atmosphere and usually produces a bean with more sophisticated flavor. Many strains of each variety have been bred and refined. At Cooper's plantation in Keauhou, we examined his *criollo* trees.

"This place is perfect for growing cacao," Bob Cooper explained to us. Cacao trees are adaptable to a wide range of moisture conditions. They can grow in zones that range from subtropical dry to tropical very wet, but they require fairly consistent temperature averaging around 26° C (79° F) for healthy growth. Cacao tolerates wind well, thrives best in high humidity and rainfall, and requires deep, well-drained soil. "When my wife, Pam, and I moved here from North Carolina in 1997, we wanted to make the best chocolate coming out of Hawaii. You just can't compare the flavor of any of the foreign-bean chocolate made here and chocolate from real Hawaiian cacao. We have six acres here, and this spot is just perfect for cacao. It loves this area, just like coffee does. These trees thrive here. And the beans get this amazingly complex flavor, like no other chocolate. Just look at these beautiful trees. We're so proud of them." We wandered through the well-maintained plantation, admiring healthy, beautiful cacao trees.

Making the Food of the Gods

Bob walked us over to an area where cocoa beans were being fermented. "See, we handpick ripe pods when they're red or maroon colored, then we slice them open. Inside each pod are beans covered with white mucilage that looks and tastes nothing like chocolate. We scoop the beans from the pods, and we ferment them in slatted wooden boxes. This is where you get the most changes in the bean. Fermentation brings out the flavor and aroma of the cacao. We get the beans down to 8 percent moisture, so they won't spoil. After the beans are fermented, we spread them out on drying racks in the sun for about twenty-five days."

I am impressed by human ingenuity when I learn about processing methods such as those required to make chocolate. Fermentation is just the first in a series of steps that include roasting, cooling, making a paste, and separating cocoa solids from the fatty cocoa butter. At that point the process is half complete. The cocoa solids are then loaded into huge grinding machines and ground into a very fine paste. Cocoa butter is reintroduced, along with sugar, lecithin, and vanilla. The amount of added butter will vary, depending on the type of chocolate being produced. Milk chocolate contains the highest amount of overall fat and only around 25 percent cocoa content. Strong, dark, semisweet chocolate may contain 75 percent cocoa solids and less butter and sugar than other chocolates.

When all the ingredients are mixed together, they are "conched," blended in large, highly specialized machines until a totally smooth, creamy, homogeneous mixture results. In the very last stage of chocolate manufacturing, the liquid material is cooled and then gently heated, to stabilize the fat crystals in the chocolate. This process gives chocolate its characteristic sheen and texture. Once tempered, the chocolate is poured and allowed to cool. The food of the gods is ready for our pleasure.

Agents of Bliss and Love

Chocolate is a complex material possessing numerous compounds that act upon the brain, producing a sense of delight that no other substance can replicate. Chocolate is surprisingly good for health, especially for the heart. Cocoa, the primary ingredient in finished chocolate, is rich in antioxidant polyphenols, a group of protective chemicals found in many plant foods including red wine and tea. The polyphenols in chocolate help to reduce the oxidation of LDL, or so-called bad cholesterol, a major risk factor in coronary disease. Additionally, polyphenols inhibit blood platelets from clumping together, reducing the risk of atherosclerosis, hardening of the arteries.

From a cardiovascular health standpoint, the very best ways to benefit from the heart-enhancing effects of chocolate are either to consume cocoa powder or to eat a moderate amount of semisweet dark chocolate. Cocoa powder can be used liberally to make hot cocoa, with milk or water and can be added to blender drinks and baked goods. Cocoa powder contains little fat and no sugar. Sweeten lightly, but keep the sugar content down. If you go the finished chocolate route, keep your consumption to about half a 3.5-ounce bar of semisweet dark chocolate daily.

Our interests here concern enhancement of mind and mood and the experience of love. In this regard, the first two compounds in chocolate to consider are caffeine and theobromine. Caffeine, an alkaloid, is the most widely consumed stimulant on earth. According to numerous medical studies caffeine is beneficial to overall health. Caffeine stimulates the central nervous system, stimulates the flow of blood in the brain, and increases secretion of the very important neurotransmitter serotonin.

Caffeine enhances alertness, facilitates thought formation, and decreases fatigue. This alkaloid also improves mood overall, lifts the spirits, and enhances both cardiovascular function and respiration.

Taken by adults at a dose of 300 milligrams or less per day, caffeine is safe and beneficial. Chocolate is a modest caffeine source, with a 50-gram piece of dark chocolate yielding between 10 and 60 milligrams of caffeine, as compared with a five-ounce cup of coffee, which can yield up to 180 milligrams. Modest amounts of caffeine in chocolate provide a healthy stimulant effect, suitable for consumption by all adults and children, except for the unusually sensitive or hyperactive. Please keep in mind that the sugar in chocolate is not suitable for diabetics.

Theobromine, caffeine's chemical cousin, occurs at a greater concentration, about 250 milligrams in a 50-gram bar of dark chocolate. Like caffeine, theobromine is a central-nervous-system stimulant, though it is milder in its effects. Theobromine is a stronger cardiac stimulant than caffeine and not nearly as well studied. This compound has a different chemical structure and is presumed to possess unique mood-enhancing effects.

Chocolate gets right to the heart of sexual pleasure by increasing the brain's level of serotonin, the feel-good brain chemical. Serotonin plays a major role in positive mood, emotional health, proper sleep, and balanced appetite, contributing to numerous behavioral and physiological functions. Decreased serotonin is a well-known factor in cases of depression. Increased brain serotonin promoted by chocolate increases sexual excitation, desire, and responsiveness. Women have more serotonin in their systems than men and appear to be more sensitive to chocolate. Chocolate provides a mood boost to women during

PMS and menstruation, when serotonin levels are often down. It also puts women in the mood for love. Men and women with depleted serotonin levels demonstrate increased aggressive sexual tendencies, a higher rate of masturbation, and increased promiscuity. Violence, aggressive behaviors, and higher rates of suicide have all been associated with reduced brain levels of serotonin. Many people consume chocolate as a form of self-medication, whether they are aware of the fact or not. Chocolate's serotonin-elevating activity helps to modify mood in positive ways and acts as a sexual sweetener, enhancing the sense of closeness between lovers.

Probably the most influential love compound in chocolate is PEA, phenethylamine. This chemical, which occurs in chocolate in small quantities, stimulates the nervous system and triggers the release of pleasurable opiumlike compounds known as endorphins. PEA also potentiates the activity of dopamine, a neurochemical directly associated with sexual arousal and pleasure. PEA acts as a potent antidepressant in both sexes and rises during periods of romance. The giddy, restless feelings that occur when we are in love are due to a great extent to PEA, which significantly increases in the brain at that time, and when we achieve orgasm. Some scientists dismiss this notion, claiming that the PEA in chocolate is metabolized too quickly to produce a significant mood-altering effect, but others disagree. Why else would chocolate be so inextricably intertwined with love and romance? While there are a great many agents in nature that boost libido and enhance sexual function, chocolate alone actually promotes the brain chemistry of being in love.

The popular drug cannabis (marijuana) contains a group of compounds called cannabinoids. Of these, THC, or tetrahydrocannabinol, causes the high associated when that plant is consumed. Cannabinoids are found in only two other places. One is in the human brain, where a mind-altering cannabinoid named anandamide is manufactured. This same extraordinary chemical is also found in chocolate. Anandamide's name derives from the Sanskrit word *ananda*, which means bliss. Cannabis and chocolate and the human brain all share this bliss-inducing agent. In the human brain, anandamide binds to the same receptor sites as THC from cannabis. Anandamide produces a feeling of euphoria. This compound may account for why some people become blissed-out when they eat chocolate. The human brain is a marvelous and mysterious organ. Tickle the right neurons with delicious chocolate, and all heaven breaks loose.

Not everybody will fall madly in love, become highly sexually aroused, or swoon with ecstatic bliss after a bite of good chocolate. Individual chemistry plays a major role in how people react to chocolate, as it does with almost everything else. Chocolate may produce a modest effect in some people, but it will make others swoon.

Venezuela Cacao

Chocolate is a lot like wine. Once you get into it, you discover that fine chocolates offer different flavors and aromas according to the origin of the beans from which they are made. In the worlds of wine and coffee we have seen a transformation from homogeneous flavors to unique varietals. It used to be that you drank red or white wine. Now you choose an Alexander Valley Cabernet, or a Napa Valley Sauvignon Blanc. With coffee, you can choose Colombian Supremo, or Kenya AA, or Sumatra Mandehling. There are many fine varieties of wines and coffees. As people's tastes become more sophisticated, they want to try new flavors. The same phenomenon is happening with chocolate. We are drifting from one-taste-fits-all bars like Hershey and Cadbury to chocolates that range from earthy to floral, bitter to sweet, light to heavy. Beans from one country result in markedly different chocolate than beans from another. Even within a small geographic region, beans can vary widely in their flavor and aroma characteristics, due to differences in soil and climate.

In the world of chocolate, probably no company understands the unique subtleties of beans from one plantation to another better than Chocolates El Rey, located in Venzuela. The entire African continent produces an impressive one million tons of cocoa beans per year, the country of Venezuela only fourteen thousand tons. Yet Venezuela produces some of the loveliest, most elegant-tasting cocoa beans on earth. Many chefs worldwide choose to use Venezuelan chocolate in their desserts and pastries. And most of the time, they choose El Rey. Timothy Moley first told me about Chocolates El Rey. "If you really want to go all the way to the heart of excellent chocolate, they're probably the best people to see." With that ringing endorsement, I booked passage to Caracas, Venezuela, for myself and my close friend Craig Weatherby. When I contacted El Rey, a man named K. C. Miller agreed to meet us and show us around.

Possessing an indomitably positive attitude, K. C. was brimming with excitement about chocolate. He also knew his way around blindfolded. A big man with a big truck and big talk, K. C. showed us the finest of northern Venezuela's cacao plantations, where the beans grew that would be transformed into the finest chocolates on earth. As we rode along K. C. gave us a crash course in the Venezuelan cacao trade and explained how El Rey's owner Jorge Redmond had created a line of chocolates that was the envy of the confectionery world. "There isn't anything Jorge won't do to make an excellent chocolate," K. C. told us. "It's just like a fine winery. Every little detail either contributes to a great product, or it takes away. So Jorge works it all the way from the plantations to the types of machines in the factory."

After nine days of scenic and informative travel throughout the Venezuelan countryside, K. C. drove Craig and me to the small city of Barquisimeto, where the Chocolates El Rey factory is located. After donning white gowns and protective nets for our hair, we were led on a tour of the manufacturing plant that left us salivating for some of the chocolate we had seen being made. "Well," K. C. told us, "I think that after lunch we're going to have us a little tasting. You're going to go nuts when you taste what we have."

After lunch K. C. sat Craig and me at a large conference table at the headquarters of Chocolates El Rey. Spread before us lay five plates piled high with different types of dark chocolate. He handed us each a scorecard with the names of the chocolates and spaces to comment on aroma, flavor, texture, and overall impression. Then K. C. poured chilled Venezuelan champagne into fluted glasses. "This is to cleanse the palate," he noted.

Our approach to the chocolate tasting was the same as the approach experts take to evaluate fine wines, coffees, or teas. We were about to engage our senses of smell and taste to sample the chocolates before us and to offer critical evaluation.

"Okay, here's what we've got here," K. C. explained. "Each of these chocolates is a seventy-percent cocoa chocolate, and each one is made from a different cacao from a different region." K. C. went on to explain that Chocolates El Rey produces varietal chocolates from cacao harvested at specific plantations, with remarkable differences in flavor and aroma.

K. C. conducted the tasting like a professor on the opening day of a science class. "This one is Macuro, from the Rio Caribe area. This one is Gran Saman, made from our special Carenero Superior cacao beans from the Barlovento area, in north central Venezuela. This one here is Apamate', also a Carenero Superior bean, but a different mix of cacao solids and cocoa butter. This one is Sur Del Lago from south of Lake Maracaibo, and this one, San Joaquin, is made from an Ocumare' bean from Barinas state. So what I recommend you do is take any kind and chew it slowly, and just let it melt in your mouth, so you can really taste the subtle flavors." Craig and I required no further urging. We picked up pieces and began tasting.

Each of the five chocolates was outstanding, but two of the samples stood out above the rest. The Gran Saman possessed complex earthy and woody flavor notes and finished with a soft, lingering bitterness. The San Joaquin narrowly won the day, possessed of a complex sweetness and a lingering smokiness. K. C. laughed when Craig and I both announced the San Joaquin as a favorite. "You can't even get that one in the States. Every kilo we make goes right to Japan." Craig and I looked at K. C. with dismay. He rushed to reassure us. "Of course, I could send you home with a few kilos." We did in fact travel home with several kilos of San Joaquin chocolate in our luggage. Mine was gone in about two months. It was the best chocolate I have ever enjoyed.

Using Chocolate

I wouldn't leave you hanging here, salivating for chocolates you can't find. You can order from Chocolates El Rey online at www.chocolates-elrey.com and from The Original Hawaiian Chocolate Factory at www.originalhawaiianchocolatefactory. com. Chocolove is available in most natural food stores and gourmet stores throughout the United States.

As I said earlier in this chapter, chocolate isn't specifically a sex herb. It is a love drug. The best way to enjoy the love-promoting effects of chocolate is with your partner. And the best time to enjoy chocolate together is before or during making love. Share a bar of the good stuff. Maybe lick it off of each other. Make a game of it, or a sensual ritual. And then do what lovers do. Get real close, and lose yourselves in each other.

I wish you all good and happy loving.

HOT PLANTS RESOURCES

As you know by now, nature offers a remarkable array of effective sex-enhancing botanicals, the hot plants I have described in the preceeding chapters. You know what they are, where they come from, and how they have been traditionally used. The hot plants can boost your libido, enhance your sexual pleasure, and improve your sexual function. The next step in our odyssey together is to put together the hot plants and other lifestyle tools, to enhance your sex life by enhancing your life overall.

In this section, I am going to introduce you to two Hot Plants formulas that combine all these marvelous natural sex enhancers together for you. And I am going to give you some information on other lifestyle factors that sabotage your sex life. Additionally, I am going to direct you to high-quality brands of individual hot plants, if you wish to use one or more of them by themselves.

For more information, visit my Web site. www. medicinehunter.com.

The Hot Plants Formulas

Early on in the writing of this book, I realized that I would serve the interests of readers best by putting the sex-enhancing botanicals I've researched into superior quality, potent formulas. This is to make it easy for you to derive the benefits of the hot plants and to ensure that superior quality products will be available in the market.

I will not denigrate other products. But I will say that I am personally very selective about which herbal brands and ingredients pass muster with me. There is tremendous variation in quality in the herbal market. The challenge for a formulator who wishes to develop effective products is to select the best-researched, purest, highest-quality and -potency raw botanicals and botanical extracts available. Many producers make cheap herbal formulas with cheap ingredients. That approach does not result in a potent, effective product. If you go out into the market searching for effective hot plants, you should be able to find them readily.

In developing the Hot Plants formulas, I have worked closely with Enzymatic Therapy of Green Bay, Wisconsin. Enzymatic, as they are commonly known, has an impeccable reputation for the quality of their supplements and excellent distribution in the marketplace. You can find their products from coast to coast. I needed a partner who would not hesitate to use very high quality botanicals. They didn't flinch at all. And I wanted you to be able to walk into any of thousands of natural products stores and obtain these formulas.

My two formulas are **Hot Plants For Him**, and **Hot Plants For Her.**

Hot Plants For Him contains horny goat weed, *Rhodiola rosea,* yohimbe, *Panax ginseng,* Tongkat Ali, and MacaPure.

Hot Plants For Her contains *Rhodiola rosea,* ashwagandha, catuaba, *Eleutherococcus senticosus,* and MacaPure.

Both formulas will start a fire in your loins. These products simplify the search for hot plants and give both men and women outstanding quality sex-enhancing herbal products in ready-to-use form, in the right doses. Both formulas are under the Enzymatic Therapy brand, and can be found all over the United States. If you can't find these Hot Plants formulas, visit the Enzymatic Therapy Web site at: www.enzy.com.

Lifestyle Factors That Sabotage Your Sex Life

Here I wish to mention a few points about three specific lifestyle factors that can sabotage your sex life. At the very top of the list is smoking cigarettes. I am continually amazed that millions of people still smoke, even after decades of high-profile information about the deadly effects of this pernicious addiction. Smoking damages circulation, respiration, and overall health. Smoking causes heart attack and stroke, and contributes to hardening of the arteries. Smoking damages blood vessels, and this can lead to reduced blood flow, reduced sensitivity, and poor erectile function. It is the leading cause of cancer, it causes birth defects, and it stinks. Recent British medical studies identify smoking as a cause of impotence. I am not saying that you cannot have a decent sex life if you smoke. But I am saying that if you smoke, you will likely wind up with health problems that will compromise your sex life, and everything else. Of all the addictions, cigarette smoking is reputedly the single most difficult to overcome. And yet many people do successfully quit and go on to live happier, healthier lives. Whatever it takes, if you are a cigarette smoker, quit. Join a program, seek help. But quit. Instead of smoking cigarettes, make love.

Overuse of alcohol is another factor that can damage your liver, brain, digestion, and sex life. Excess alcohol consumption can lead to esophageal inflammation and cancer, gastritis, ulcers, pancreatic inflammation and cancer, abnormal heartbeat and heart failure, high blood pressure, atherosclerosis, stroke, confusion, reduced memory, and deterioration of nerves in the arms and legs. If you drink more than moderately, cut back. If you cannot cut back on your own, seek help. Our sexual vitality is representative of our overall vitality and health. If you are consuming too much alcohol, which is a sedative-hypnotic drug, then you will debilitate yourself. If you are sapped from booze, you will have little sexual vitality for living.

The same goes for drug abuse. By this I don't mean smoking a little pot, which is a benign habit from every known health standpoint. Cocaine, amphetamines, barbiturates, heroin, and other potent drugs can and will mess you up, and render you sexually disinterested and incapable. In the United States, we have a huge problem with hard drug abuse. From alcohol, the gateway drug, people often go on to other dangerous drugs, ruining themselves and creating havoc among family and friends. When you are a drug abuser, the happy pleasures of satisfying sex are usually supplanted by drug cravings and disorientation. As with alcohol, if you are abusing these classes of drugs, seek help.

If you want to maintain a healthy sex life for a long time, you need to maintain overall health. Eliminating blatantly destructive, enervating habits is one way to boost your overall health and vitality, ensuring a more dynamic sex life in the bargain.

Lifestyle Factors That Enhance Your Sex Life

A multitude of factors influence our sex lives. One common problem that many people face is making too little time for life's pleasures, including sex. This is a mistake. The very best thing for your sex life is having regular sex. There really is something to the expression "use it or lose it." Enjoying regular sex keeps you active and stimulated, and will create a source of ongoing pleasure. Infrequent sex reduces your overall pleasure and sense of satisfaction. Life's pleasures, especially sex, are meant to be enjoyed. Each of us is equipped with elaborate pleasure mechanisms. These exist so that we can derive maximum pleasure from a variety of experiences. Pleasure is essential to a happy life, and pleasure is associated with sexual activity.

I know that the advice I just gave may prove difficult for some people to follow, especially if you are living a high-stress lifestyle. As I have discussed in previous chapters, stress causes innumerable flaccid erections, dry vaginas, and cases of lost sexual desire in men and women. We come under physical, emotional, and mental stress from many situations and circumstances. Stress causes biochemical damage that can result in reduced sexual desire and impaired sexual function in men and women. A few of the hot plants, notably *Rhodiola rosea,* ashwagandha, and *Eleutherococcus senticosus,* combat the effects of stress upon the body and mind. Taking them can be a significant step toward sexual reinvigoration.

Finding the Hot Plants

If you wish to find the individual hot plants, the following are products of high quality, with assured potency. You will find most of these brands in good natural food stores. If you cannot find them in stores near you, then the associated Web sites, which are also given here, will prove helpful. For your convenience, I have listed the hot plants and their sources in order of appearance in the text.

I have described the use and effects of the hot plants throughout the book and am not going to repeat those points here. But you may wonder whether you can use the hot plants in combination with each other. The answer is yes. That is why I developed the Hot Plants formulas. Traditionally, plants are often used together in combination.

I recommend that you either use the Hot Plants formulas, or you try individual hot plants one at a time. You may find that simply taking Tongkat Ali or maca or *Rhodiola rosea* is sufficient to boost your libido and enhance sexual function. Keep in mind that these are not like synthetic drugs. An herb may take several days or a couple of weeks to produce the effects you seek.

If you are under a lot of stress, the adaptogens *Rhodiola rosea,* ashwagandha, *Eleutherococcus senticosus,* and *Panax ginseng* are for you. Otherwise, finding the right hot plant for you may require some experimentation. I have given you plenty of information about the effects and uses of these herbs.

TONGKAT ALI

The company that has rights to U.S. distribution of the LJ100 Tongkat Ali extract I have written about is Herbal Powers. You can obtain LJ100 by ordering from their Web site or by phone. http://www.herbal-powers.com

Order by Phone: 1-866-330-HERB, ext. 1

The other company that sells LJ100 Tongkat Ali extract is Source Naturals, whose products are distributed through natural food stores. Look for their Tongkat Ali Male Libido Tonic.
http://www.sourcenaturals.com

RHODIOLA ROSEA
I will recommend four *Rhodiola rosea* products for you.

Yellow Emperor
You will most likely have to order by Web or phone. Yellow Emperor's fluid extract product Siberian *Rhodiola Rosea* comes in a liquid spray, and is very fast acting.
http://www.yellowemperor.com

Pinnacle
Another very fine *Rhodiola rosea* product is Rhodax, made by Pinnacle products. You can find Rhodax in most GNC stores and in other natural food stores.
http://www.pinnaclebody.com

New Chapter
New Chapter labels its *Rhodiola rosea* capsules Rhodiola. You can find New Chapter products in natural food stores.
http://www.new-chapter.com

Enzymatic Therapy
Enzymatic calls their product Rhodiola Energy. You can find Enzymatic Therapy products in natural food stores.
http://www.enzy.com

YOHIMBE

Twin Lab

You will find Twin Lab Yohimbe Fuel in GNC stores and natural foods stores.

http://www.twinlab.com

Ultimate Nutrition

This division of Nutraceutical Corp makes a standardized yohimbe tablet product, Yohimbe Bark Extract, available in natural food stores.

http://www.nutraceutical.com

HORNY GOAT WEED

The horny goat weed formula I described in this book is made by Pinnacle products. It is called simply Horny Goat Weed. This is the formula that has proven successful in human clinical studies.

http://www.pinnaclebody.com

ASHWAGANDHA

Planetary Formulas

This company makes an Ashwagandha Liquid Herbal Extract. You can find Planetary Formulas products in natural food stores.

http://www.planetaryformulas.com

Nature's Herbs

Distributed throughout natural food stores, Nature's Herbs makes a tableted Ashwagandha.

http://www.naturesherbs.com

CATUABA

For catuaba products, see Raintree Nutrition. You will have to order by Web or phone. Perusing the Raintree Web site is a door-opener into another world. Excellent.
http://www.rain-tree.com

ZALLOUH

Nutranex, the primary company I knew of that sold zallouh root, went out of business after I began writing *Hot Plants*. The Internet offers a plethora of zallouh-based products, but I cannot vouch for any of them, due to lack of familiarity. Thus, with zallouh root you are on your own. I am confident that zallouh, with its history of safe and very effective use, will come on strong in the marketplace over time. But as of now, you will have to do a bit of experimenting to find a source that delivers.

MACA

The maca extract I know to be absolutely superior to all other maca products is MacaPure, which is standardized to 0.6 percent Macamides and Macaenes. GNC sells a standardized maca product that is MacaPure, without listing the MacaPure name. Look for any maca product that says it is standardized to 0.6 percent Macamides and Macaenes. This will be MacaPure.

Vimaca

A product called Vimaca (one for men, one for women) also contains MacaPure. You will find Vimaca on the Web.
http://www.vimaca.com

NutraMedix

If you are willing to toss a spoonful of maca powder into a

blender drink (it's good), buy the 4-ounce container of powdered maca from NutraMedix.
http://nutramedix.com

ELEUTHEROCOCCUS SENTICOSUS

Nature's Way
    This popular herb company makes Siberian Eleuthero Root Extract capsules, found in natural food stores.
http://naturesway.com

Superior Trading Company
    This leader in eleuthero and panax ginseng products offers single-serve ampules of fluid Eleuthero Ginseng Extract, available in natural food stores.
http://www.superiortrading.com

PANAX GINSENG

Superior Trading Company
    This leader in eleuthero and panax ginseng products offers single-serve ampules of fluid Red Panax Ginseng Extractum, available in natural food stores.
http://www.superiortrading.com

Also, look for the Pines brand of Chinese ginseng extract products, available in natural food stores, and in Chinese herbal stores and groceries.

Also, see the Prince Of Peace Web site for a plethora of Eleuthero and Panax ginseng products, all good.
http://www.popus.com